T0226532

PET/MRI: Advances in Instrumentation and Quantitative Procedures

Editor

HABIB ZAIDI

PET CLINICS

www.pet.theclinics.com

Consulting Editor
ABASS ALAVI

April 2016 • Volume 11 • Number 2

ELSEVIER

1600 John F. Kennedy Boulevard • Suite 1800 • Philadelphia, Pennsylvania, 19103-2899

http://www.pet.theclinics.com

PET CLINICS Volume 11, Number 2
April 2016 ISSN 1556-8598, ISBN-13: 978-0-323-41767-9

Editor: John Vassallo (j.vassallo@elsevier.com)
Developmental Editor: Meredith Clinton

PET Clinics (ISSN 1556-8598) is published quarterly by Elsevier Inc., 360 Park Avenue South, New York, NY 10010-1710. Months of issue are January, April, July, and October. Periodicals postage paid at New York, NY, and additional mailing offices. Subscription prices per year are $225.00 (US individuals), $366.00 (US institutions), $100.00 (US students), $255.00 (Canadian individuals), $412.00 (Canadian institutions), $140.00 (Canadian students), $260.00 (foreign individuals), $412.00 (foreign institutions), and $140.00 (foreign students). To receive student and resident rate, orders must be accompanied by name of affiliated institution, date of term, and the signature of program/residency coordinator on institution letterhead. Orders will be billed at individual rate until proof of status is received. Foreign air speed delivery is included in all Clinics subscription prices. All prices are subject to change without notice. POSTMASTER: Send address changes to PET Clinics, Elsevier Health Sciences Division, Subscription Customer Service, 3251 Riverport Lane, Maryland Heights, MO 63043. **Customer Service: 1-800-654-2452 (U.S. and Canada); 314-447-8871 (outside U.S. and Canada). Fax: 314-447-8029. E-mail: journalscustomerservice-usa@elsevier.com (for print support); journalsonlinesupport-usa@elsevier.com (for online support).**

Reprints. For copies of 100 or more of articles in this publication, please contact the Commercial Reprints Department, Elsevier Inc., 360 Park Avenue South, New York, NY 10010-1710. Tel.: 212-633-3874; Fax: 212-633-3820; E-mail: reprints@elsevier.com.

PET Clinics is covered in MEDLINE/PubMed (Index Medicus).

Contributors

CONSULTING EDITOR

ABASS ALAVI, MD, PhD (Hon), Dsc (Hon)
Professor of Radiology, Division of Nuclear
Medicine, Department of Radiology, University
of Pennsylvania School of Medicine, Hospital
of the University of Pennsylvania, Philadelphia,
Pennsylvania

EDITOR

HABIB ZAIDI, PhD
Division of Nuclear Medicine and Molecular
Imaging, Geneva University Hospital, Geneva,
Switzerland

AUTHORS

SIMON ARRIDGE, PhD
Department of Computer Science,
University College London, London,
United Kingdom

DAVID ATKINSON, PhD
Centre for Medical Imaging, University
College London, London, United Kingdom

JASON BINI, PhD
Department of Diagnostic Radiology, PET
Center, Yale School of Medicine, Yale
University, New Haven, Connecticut

CIPRIAN CATANA, MD, PhD
Assistant Professor, Department of Radiology,
Athinoula A. Martinos Center for Biomedical
Imaging, Massachusetts General Hospital,
Harvard Medical School, Charlestown,
Massachusetts

RAFAEL T.M. DE ROSALES, PhD
Division of Imaging Sciences and
Biomedical Engineering, King's College
London, St. Thomas' Hospital, London,
United Kingdom

JOHN DICKSON, PhD
Institute of Nuclear Medicine, University
College London Hospital, London, United
Kingdom

MOOTAZ ELDIB, MS
Translational and Molecular Imaging
Institute, Icahn School of Medicine at
Mount Sinai; Department of Biomedical
Engineering, The City College of New York,
New York, New York

KJELL ERLANDSSON, PhD
Institute of Nuclear Medicine, University
College London, London, United Kingdom

DAVID D. FAUL, PhD
Siemens Healthcare, New York, New York

ZAHI A. FAYAD, PhD
Director, Translational and Molecular
Imaging Institute; Department of Radiology;
Department of Cardiology, Zena and
Michael A. Weiner Cardiovascular Institute,
Marie-Josée and Henry R. Kravis
Cardiovascular Health Center; Icahn School of
Medicine at Mount Sinai, New York, New York

JÉRÉMIE P. FOUQUET, BSc
Department of Nuclear Medicine and
Radiobiology, Centre d'imagerie moléculaire
de Sherbrooke (CIMS), Université de
Sherbrooke, Sherbrooke, Québec, Canada

HANS HERZOG, PhD
Institute of Neuroscience and Medicine – 4,
Forschungszentrum Jülich, Jülich, Germany

BRIAN F. HUTTON, PhD
Institute of Nuclear Medicine, University
College London, London, United Kingdom; The
Centre for Medical Radiation Physics,
University of Wollongong, Wollongong,
Australia

DAVID IZQUIERDO-GARCIA, PhD
Instructor, Department of Radiology,
Athinoula A. Martinos Center for Biomedical
Imaging, Massachusetts General Hospital,
Harvard Medical School, Charlestown,
Massachusetts

CHRISTOPH KOLBITSCH, PhD
Research Associate, Division of Imaging
Sciences and Biomedical Engineering,
Department of Biomedical Engineering, King's
College London, St. Thomas' Hospital,
London, United Kingdom

RÉJEAN LEBEL, PhD
Department of Nuclear Medicine and
Radiobiology, Centre d'imagerie moléculaire
de Sherbrooke (CIMS), Université de
Sherbrooke, Sherbrooke, Québec, Canada

MARTIN LEPAGE, PhD
Department of Nuclear Medicine and
Radiobiology, Centre d'imagerie moléculaire
de Sherbrooke (CIMS), Université de
Sherbrooke, Sherbrooke, Québec, Canada

CHRISTOPH LERCHE, PhD
Institute of Neuroscience and Medicine – 4,
Forschungszentrum Jülich, Jülich, Germany

GEORGE LOUDOS, PhD
Assistant Professor, Department of Biomedical
Engineering, Technological Educational
Institute of Athens, Athens, Greece

PAUL MARSDEN, PhD
Professor, Division of Imaging Sciences and
Biomedical Engineering, Department of
Biomedical Engineering, King's College
London, St. Thomas' Hospital, London,
United Kingdom

CAMILA MUNOZ, MSc
PhD Student, Division of Imaging Sciences and
Biomedical Engineering, Department of
Biomedical Engineering, King's College
London, St. Thomas' Hospital, London,
United Kingdom

NIELS OESINGMANN, PhD
Siemens Healthcare, New York, New York

SEBASTIEN OURSELIN, PhD
Centre for Medical Imaging Computing,
University College London, London,
United Kingdom

CLAUDIA PRIETO, PhD
Lecturer, Division of Imaging Sciences and
Biomedical Engineering, Department of
Biomedical Engineering, King's College
London, St. Thomas' Hospital, London,
United Kingdom

ANDREW J. READER, PhD
Reader, Division of Imaging Sciences and
Biomedical Engineering, Department of
Biomedical Engineering, King's College
London, St. Thomas' Hospital, London,
United Kingdom

MARIE ANNE RICHARD, BSc
Department of Nuclear Medicine and
Radiobiology, Centre d'imagerie moléculaire
de Sherbrooke (CIMS), Université de
Sherbrooke, Sherbrooke, Québec, Canada

LYDIA SANDIFORD, PhD
Division of Imaging Sciences and Biomedical
Engineering, King's College London, St.
Thomas' Hospital, London, United Kingdom

TOBIAS SCHAEFFTER, PhD
Professor, Division of Imaging Sciences and
Biomedical Engineering, Department of
Biomedical Engineering, King's College
London, St. Thomas' Hospital, London,
United Kingdom

CHARALAMPOS TSOUMPAS, PhD
Translational and Molecular Imaging
Institute, Icahn School of Medicine at
Mount Sinai, New York, New York;
Lecturer, Division of Biomedical Imaging,
Faculty of Medicine and Health,
University of Leeds, Leeds,
United Kingdom

DIMITRIS VISVIKIS, PhD
Professor, LaTIM UMR 1101, INSERM,
University of Brest, Brest, France

Contents

approaches and their pros and cons. The main sources of artifacts are presented. Finally, this review discusses the current status of MR-AC approaches for clinical applications.

With the introduction of clinical PET/magnetic resonance (MR) systems, novel attenuation correction methods are needed, as there are no direct MR methods to measure the attenuation of the objects in the field of view (FOV). A unique challenge for PET/MR attenuation correction is that coils for MR data acquisition are located in the FOV of the PET camera and could induce significant quantitative errors. In this review, current methods and techniques to correct for the attenuation of a variety of coils are summarized and evaluated.

Partial volume effects are caused by the limited spatial resolution of the PET system. There is increasing evidence that partial volume correction (PVC) is necessary to guarantee quantitative accuracy in PET; however, there is reluctance to apply PVC routinely in clinical practice, partly because of uncertainty regarding the method of choice. To perform accurate PVC, it is necessary to introduce information from high-resolution anatomic images, such as MR imaging. All the methods rely on accurate coregistration between the anatomic image and the PET image. PET/MR imaging offers clear advantages for PVC and can help alleviate the image registration issues.

Cardiac and respiratory motion cause image quality degradation in PET imaging, affecting diagnostic accuracy of the images. Whole-body simultaneous PET-MR scanners allow for using motion information estimated from MR images to correct PET data and produce motion-compensated PET images. This article reviews methods that have been proposed to estimate motion from MR images and different techniques to include this information in PET reconstruction, in order to overcome the problem of cardiac and respiratory motion in PET-MR imaging. MR-based motion correction techniques significantly increase lesion detectability and contrast, and also improve accuracy of uptake values in PET images.

Blood samples obtained by arterial cannulation are the gold standard to measure the input function for PET pharmacokinetic modeling. There is interest in less invasive methods, such as image-derived input functions (IDAIF). MRI can be used to segment and correct partial volume effects of the PET images, improving IDAIF extraction. Preclinical studies have shown that the input function of PET tracers, namely fluorodeoxyglucose and [^{18}F]fluoroethyl-L-tyrosine, can be derived from the Gd-DTPA input function. Noninvasive, MRI-guided, PET input function derivation is a promising avenue to reduce or eliminate the need for arterial plasma samples in preclinical and clinical settings.

PET CLINICS

PROGRAM OBJECTIVE

The goal of the *PET Clinics* is to keep practicing radiologists and radiology residents up to date with current clinical practice in positron emission tomography by providing timely articles reviewing the state of the art in patient care.

TARGET AUDIENCE

Practicing radiologists, radiology residents, and other health care professionals who provide patient care utilizing radiologic findings.

LEARNING OBJECTIVES

Upon completion of this activity, participants will be able to:
1. Review advances in the clinical implementation of MRI and PET.
2. Discuss methods of using contrast agents in clinical and pre-clinical PET-MRI.
3. Recognize innovations in MR-based correction for motion and positron emission tomography data in PET-MR imaging.

ACCREDITATION

The Elsevier Office of Continuing Medical Education (EOCME) is accredited by the Accreditation Council for Continuing Medical Education (ACCME) to provide continuing medical education for physicians.

The EOCME designates this enduring material for a maximum of 15 *AMA PRA Category 1 Credit*(s)™. Physicians should claim only the credit commensurate with the extent of their participation in the activity.

All other health care professionals requesting continuing education credit for this enduring material will be issued a certificate of participation.

DISCLOSURE OF CONFLICTS OF INTEREST

The EOCME assesses conflict of interest with its instructors, faculty, planners, and other individuals who are in a position to control the content of CME activities. All relevant conflicts of interest that are identified are thoroughly vetted by EOCME for fair balance, scientific objectivity, and patient care recommendations. EOCME is committed to providing its learners with CME activities that promote improvements or quality in healthcare and not a specific proprietary business or a commercial interest.

The planning committee, staff, authors and editors listed below have identified no financial relationships or relationships to products or devices they or their spouse/life partner have with commercial interest related to the content of this CME activity:

Abass Alavi, MD, PhD (Hon), Dsc (Hon); Simon Arridge, PhD; David Atkinson, PhD; Jason Bini, PhD; Ciprian Catana, MD, PhD; Rafael T.M. de Rosales, PhD; John Dickson, PhD; Mootaz Eldib, MS; Kjell Erlandsson, PhD; Zahi A. Fayad, PhD; Anjali Fortna; Jérémie P. Fouquet, BSc; Hans Herzog, PhD; Brian F. Hutton, PhD; David Izquierdo-Garcia, PhD; Christoph Kolbitsch, PhD; Réjean Lebel, PhD; Martin Lepage, PhD; Christoph Lerche, PhD; George Loudos, PhD; Paul Marsden, PhD; Camila Munoz, MSc; Mahalakshmi Narayanan; Sebastien Ourselin, PhD; Claudia Prieto, PhD; Andrew J. Reader, PhD; Marie Anne Richard, BSc; Lydia Sandiford, PhD; Tobias Schaeffter, PhD; Erin Scheckenbach; Charalampos Tsoumpas, PhD; John Vassallo; Dimitris Visvikis, PhD; Habib Zaidi, PhD.

The planning committee, staff, authors and editors listed below have identified financial relationships or relationships to products or devices they or their spouse/life partner have with commercial interest related to the content of this CME activity:

David D. Faul, PhD has stock ownership in, and an employment affiliation with, Siemens AG.
Niels Oesingmann, PhD is consultant/advisor for, has stock ownership in, has an employment affiliation with, and receives royalties/patents from Siemens AG.

UNAPPROVED/OFF-LABEL USE DISCLOSURE

The EOCME requires CME faculty to disclose to the participants:
1. When products or procedures being discussed are off-label, unlabelled, experimental, and/or investigational (not US Food and Drug Administration [FDA] approved); and
2. Any limitations on the information presented, such as data that are preliminary or that represent ongoing research, interim analyses, and/or unsupported opinions. Faculty may discuss information about pharmaceutical agents that is outside of FDA-approved labelling. This information is intended solely for CME and is not intended to promote off-label use of these medications. If you have any questions, contact the medical affairs department of the manufacturer for the most recent prescribing information.

TO ENROLL

To enroll in the *PET Clinics* Continuing Medical Education program, call customer service at 1-800-654-2452 or sign up online at http://www.theclinics.com/home/cme. The CME program is available to subscribers for an additional annual fee of USD $235.

METHOD OF PARTICIPATION

In order to claim credit, participants must complete the following:
1. Complete enrolment as indicated above.

2. Read the activity.
3. Complete the CME Test and Evaluation. Participants must achieve a score of 70% on the test. All CME Tests and Evaluations must be completed online.

CME INQUIRIES/SPECIAL NEEDS

For all CME inquiries or special needs, please contact elsevierCME@elsevier.com.

Preface

PET/MR Imaging: Advances in Instrumentation and Quantitative Procedures

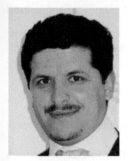

Habib Zaidi, PhD

Editor

This is an exciting time for hybrid imaging, where the success of the combination of molecular information provided by PET and structural information provided by radiographic computed tomography (CT) motivated the combination of PET with other imaging modalities, such as MR imaging, ultrasound, optical imaging, and a few other diagnostic imaging techniques. There are some interesting lessons to be learned from the history of multimodality imaging. A number of pioneers in radiological sciences realized very early (during the 1950s to 1960s) the potential and both technical and clinical benefits of combined emission and transmission imaging.[1–3] In most of the situations, the clinical demand triggered technical developments of software- and hardware-based integration of various imaging modalities to respond to this need to address clinical questions. This fact explains the widespread adoption of image coregistration software, particularly in brain imaging, and integrated whole-body PET-CT scanners, which replaced stand-alone PET scanners, in clinical oncology. The rapid pace of hybrid imaging technology has been inspired by the desire of radiologists and nuclear medicine physicians to improve over existing state-of-the-art single-modality techniques in terms of clinical diagnosis, staging and restaging, therapy response monitoring, and radiation therapy treatment planning.[4]

The history of PET/MR imaging was an exception in the sense that the emergence of this hybrid imaging modality was driven by technology and the need to address many interesting and challenging scientific questions to make the combination of the two imaging modalities possible from the instrumentation perspective, whereas the clinical applications remained unexplored and not yet established. Indeed, during the last decade, a large number of publications reported on innovative developments in MR-compatible PET detectors and various strategies to reduce the interference between the two imaging modalities. Physicists had also to rethink the issue of attenuation correction and address the many challenges of MR imaging–guided attenuation correction, particularly in whole-body PET/MR imaging. As such, this technology was regarded as "a solution looking for a problem"[5] rather than a solution to an existing problem. Indeed, despite much worthwhile research and development efforts focusing on solving technical issues, the success of any medical imaging modality is not measured by the degree of technical complexity and innovation aspect that led to its maturity.[6] It is rather measured by the sensible advantages and potential clinical benefits that this technology is going to bring in the clinical setting, keeping in mind that these have to be weighed against the substantial increase in costs and complexity for its implementation in clinical routine.

This issue of *PET Clinics* addresses the subject of hybrid PET/MR imaging technology, covering advances in both instrumentation and quantitative imaging procedures developed to address the

PET Clin 11 (2016) xiii–xiv
http://dx.doi.org/10.1016/j.cpet.2015.11.001
1556-8598/16/$ – see front matter © 2016 Published by Elsevier Inc.

above described challenges. Following the initial introduction and current commercial availability of this technology from the main leading players, offering different platforms for sequential and simultaneous PET/MR imaging, the role and limitations of this modality in clinical setting are being debated, particularly for applications in cardiology and oncology. Overall, there is a wide consensus that while this technology is still in its infancy and did not reach the required level of maturity for widespread clinical adoption, it is considered a promising advance that seems to have the potential to overcome some of the deficiencies of existing hybrid imaging modalities. During the next decade, additional exciting technical developments are foreseen and large-scale multicenter clinical trials are expected to answer critical questions regarding the clinical benefits of this technology.

In this issue of *PET Clinics*, a number of pertinent areas anticipated to play a pivotal role and have a substantial impact on the future of PET/MR imaging are highlighted. This includes advanced topics in preclinical and clinical PET/MR instrumentation and dual-modality contrast agents, MR imaging–guided partial volume and attenuation correction, including strategies to compensate for attenuation from rigid and nonrigid MR coils, as well as advanced MR imaging protocols for improved derivation of the arterial input function for PET kinetic modeling applications. It is hoped that this collection of comprehensive topics in hybrid PET/MR imaging will be useful to readers interested in both instrumentation and quantitative imaging protocols as well as their applications in clinical and research settings.

Habib Zaidi, PhD
Division of Nuclear Medicine
and Molecular Imaging
Geneva University Hospital
CH-1211 Geneva, Switzerland

E-mail address:
habib.zaidi@hcuge.ch

REFERENCES

1. Mayneord WV. The radiology of the human body with radioactive isotopes. Br J Radiol 1952;25:517–25.
2. Kuhl DE, Hale J, Eaton WL. Transmission scanning: a useful adjunct to conventional emission scanning for accurately keying isotope deposition to radiographic anatomy. Radiology 1966;87:278–84.
3. Anger HO, McRae J. Transmission scintiphotography. J Nucl Med 1968;9:267–9.
4. Torigian DA, Zaidi H, Kwee TC, et al. PET/MR imaging: technical aspects and potential clinical applications. Radiology 2013;267:26–44.
5. Yankeelov TE, Peterson TE, Abramson RG, et al. Simultaneous PET-MRI in oncology: a solution looking for a problem? Magn Reson Imaging 2012;30:1342–56.
6. Wehrl HF, Sauter AW, Divine MR, et al. Combined PET/MR: a technology becomes mature. J Nucl Med 2015;56:165–8.

Advances in Clinical PET/MRI Instrumentation

Hans Herzog, PhD*, Christoph Lerche, PhD

KEYWORDS

- Positron emission tomography • Magnetic resonance imaging • PET • MRI
- PET/MR • MRI/PET • APD • SiPM

KEY POINTS

- Five years after the installation of first whole-body PET/MRI scanners there are two simultaneous and one sequential PET/MRI systems on the market.
- The PET component of the sequential PET/MRI system is equipped with photomultiplier tubes (PMTs) and allows time-of-flight (TOF) acquisition.
- The integrated, simultaneously measuring PET/MRI scanners use avalanche photodiodes (APDs) or silicon photomultipliers (SiPMs) as readout electronics of the PET detector.
- The fast timing behavior of SiPMs allows TOF acquisition.
- The MRI component of PET/MRI is improved by dedicated sequences and coils.

INTRODUCTION

PET is an imaging diagnostic tool to observe metabolic and physiologic processes of organs in their normal and diseased states. Although PET delivers images of high radiotracer contrast, its ability to show anatomic details is limited. Therefore, the complementary use of PET with CT or MRI has been becoming common practice, which was facilitated by dedicated programs allowing the combined computer-assisted display and analysis of images acquired from different modalities.[1,2] The advantages of the combined analysis of PET and CT led to the development of hybrid scanners combining the two modalities in a single device.[3,4] The success of PET/CT scanners, especially in oncological diagnosis, led subsequently to the disappearance of PET-only scanners. On the other hand, with the continuous progress of MRI, it became clear that in comparison with CT, MRI has a superior delineation of most anatomic structures. Furthermore, today MRI not only delivers detailed anatomic information but also offers an increasing number of sequences for functional and physiologic imaging. Thus, the combination of PET and MRI in one scanner allows a one-stop-shop investigation delivering the metabolic data with PET and versatile MRI data. In addition, unlike CT, MRI does not cause a dose by ionizing radiation.

The first concept studies proving a successful combined PET/MRI measurement were performed by the group of Cherry and Marsden in 1996.[5] In the following years, different solutions were developed, at first toward simultaneous small animal PET/MRI and later toward human PET/MRI, so that in 2010 the first commercial whole-body PET/MRI system could be installed at clinical sites. This review outlines how the technical challenges of PET/MRI were solved and gives an overview of the present clinical PET/MRI equipment as

Disclosures: The authors have nothing to disclose.
Institute of Neuroscience and Medicine – 4, Forschungszentrum Jülich, Jülich 52425, Germany
* Corresponding author.
E-mail address: h.herzog@fz-juelich.de

PET Clin 11 (2016) 95–103
http://dx.doi.org/10.1016/j.cpet.2015.09.001

well as recent instrumental and methodological developments.

THE PRIMARY PROBLEMS IN COMBINING PET AND MRI AND THEIR SOLUTIONS

The major problem in the development of a single integrated PET/MRI device was that the classic readout electronics of PET detectors, the PMTs, could not be operated in the magnetic field of the MRI. Therefore, a totally new PET detector technology had to be developed. The PMTs were replaced by solid-state components that are not sensitive to magnetic fields. For this purpose, APDs were studied by Pichler and coworkers.[6] A first simultaneous PET/MRI system for small animal imaging was developed in Cherry's group that coupled an 8 × 8 array of lutetium oxyorthosilicate (LSO) crystals to a position-sensitive APD with short optical fibers of approximately 15 cm length and placed the PET detector in a Bruker BioSpec animal 7T MRI system.[7] Later, Pichler's group[8] at Tübingen University (Germany) coupled an array of LSO crystals directly to an array of single APDs and operated this magnetic-insensitive PET detector successfully within a small animal 7T MRI scanner. The PET detectors were housed in copper shielding to avoid the influence of the high-frequency MR field. Pichler's group could demonstrate that their small animal PET/MRI delivers high-quality multiparametric imaging.[9,10]

To prepare the development of an integrated whole-body PET/MRI, Siemens (Erlangen, Germany) built a prototype of a PET/MRI scanner for human brain imaging. Similar to the design proposed by Pichler and colleagues[11] the LSO crystals with a size of 2.5 × 2.5 × 20 mm³ were coupled without optical fibers to APDs. The PET ring consists of 32 copper-shielded cassettes, housing 6 detector blocks each, and was constructed as a removable insert matching the bore of a Siemens MAGNETOM Trio 3T MRI scanner. Each cassette was linked by a 10-m long shielded cable via the filter plate of the MR cabin to the data acquisition system. Because of the temperature sensitivity of the APDs, the temperature of the PET detectors was stabilized with cooled air. Within the PET ring, with its inner diameter of 36 cm, two dedicated head coils for MRI were positioned, one outer birdcage coil for combined transmittal and receiving, and one inner 8-channel coil for receiving. To test the feasibility of this new design four prototypes of the 3T MR-BrainPET scanner were installed by Siemens and evaluated in two German and two US research groups.[12–15] It could be shown that there were no remarkable interferences between the PET and the MR components. Such

interferences might have been caused by the rapidly changing MR gradient fields, inducing eddy currents in the shielding of the PET cassettes and provoking temperature increases as well as inhomogeneities of the B0 field. Another challenge was caused by the head coils, which were located between the patient's head and the PET detector, thereby attenuating the radiation emitted by the radiotracer. Therefore, the head coils were newly constructed to minimize their attenuation properties. Two of these neuro-PET/MRI scanners, which have an optimal central resolution of 3 mm, are still successfully operated by the Forschungszentrum Jülich (Jülich, Germany) and the Massachusetts General Hospital (Boston, USA).[16] Based on the experiences with the 3T MR-BrainPET and using a similar design, Siemens developed a PET/MRI system, called Biograph mMR, for simultaneous whole-body imaging.

The problem that PMTs cannot be operated in the MR field led Philips (Best, The Netherlands) to develop a sequential PET/MRI system. Because of the sequential construction no basic new instrumental developments were necessary for this scanner. The PET detector still used PMTs as readout electronics instead of APDs. To eliminate any residual influence of the MR field, the ring of PET detectors and the detectors themselves with their PMTs were shielded additionally. The PET and MRI are aligned on a common axis with a distance of 4.2 m between the centers of the fields of view (FOVs). They are coupled by a common turntable-based patient bed so that the patient can be moved quickly from one component to the other without repositioning.

CLINICAL PET/MRI INSTRUMENTATION
Sequential PET/MRI

In spring 2010, Philips was the first company to install a PET/MRI scanner for whole-body imaging: the Ingenuity TF PET/MR scanner.[17] This sequential hybrid scanner combined two well-established systems, the Philips Achieva 3T MRI scanner and the TOF-PET component of Philips Gemini PET/CT scanner. The technical specifications of the PET detector are identical to those of the Gemini TF PET/CT scanner[18]: the detector ring consists of 28 modules, each including 23 × 44 crystals made of lutetium yttrium orthosilicate (LYSO) with a size of 4 × 4 × 22 mm³. The coincidence window is set to a width of 6 nanoseconds (ns) and the energy window to 460 keV to 665 keV. The timing resolution of the TOF-PET is 525 picoseonds (ps). The axial extension of the FOV of the PET is 18 cm and that of the MRI 45 cm. The sensitivity of the PET ring is 7.2 kcps/MBq (according to the National Electrical

Manufacturers Association [NEMA] NU 2-2007 protocol[19] at r = 10 cm). A detailed description and performance evaluation of the Ingenuity TF PET/MR was published by Zaidi and colleagues.[20] Since the first installation, no instrumental upgrades of the Ingenuity TF PET/MR have been reported. Currently, approximately 10 Ingenuity TF PET/MR are installed worldwide. A first overview of experiences with this system was presented by Kalemis and colleagues.[21]

In PET/CT, the PET components of most manufacturers offer TOF performance. TOF-PET had been suggested during the early days of PET more than 30 years ago by Mullani and colleagues,[22] when they designed a PET detector with cesium fluoride scintillators, which have a very fast time resolution. Because the cesium fluoride detector showed a low sensitivity, however, they were no longer pursued and were replaced by bismuth germanium oxide (BGO) detectors, which enabled a high sensitivity but were too slow for TOF-PET. Nowadays, the PET detectors of PET/CT are equipped with LSO or LYSO scintillators. These scintillators are fast enough and – with a time resolution of, for example, 500 ps – allow TOF-PET. With TOF detection, the location of the positron emission along the line of response (LOR) can be better defined. The unknown activity to be reconstructed along an LOR is reduced by the quotient of the subject's cross-section and the width of TOF length.[23] The signal-to-noise ratio is decreased proportional to the square root of this quotient. The Ingenuity TF PET/MR can use these advantages, because the PMTs of the PET component allow fast timing, as known from present PET/CT.

The sequential combination of PET and MRI may be regarded as disadvantageous, because the study takes longer than a simultaneous one. On the other hand, PET and MRI can be acquired independently, so that the protocol of the MRI sequences does not need to be adapted to the PET protocol with its duration of 3 to 5 minutes per bed position.[24]

Like the PET/MRI scanners of other manufacturers, the Ingenuity TF PET/MR does not offer an attenuation correction (AC) based on transmission measurements as known from PET-only scanners or from PET/CT scanners. In contrast to CT, there is no relationship between the MR image intensity and the attenuation coefficient valid for photon radiation of 511 keV. Therefore, different approaches to derive attenuation maps for PET from MR images have been developed and are discussed together with related problems and possible solutions in the article by Izquierdo and Catana.[25]

The MR imaging–based AC of the Ingenuity TF PET/MR applies a specific 3-D multistack spoiled T1-weighted gradient-echo sequence, which takes approximately 3.5 minutes for a scan of 120 cm length.[26–28] The resulting image is segmented into 3 tissue classes: air, lung, and soft tissue. Because the PET and MRI acquisitions are separate, MRI coils positioned on a patient's body can be removed during the PET study so that they cause no additional attenuation.

Avalanche Photodiodes–Based PET/MRI

In November 2010, the Biograph mMR, the whole-body PET/MR of Siemens, was installed in Munich (Germany) and operated as a common project of the Technical University Munich and the Ludwig Maximilians University. This hybrid scanner allows for simultaneous measurements of PET and MRI, because the PET detector is integrated within the MRI, that is, between the gradient and the radio-frequency (RF) coils. Thus, the PET detector is not visible from outside the MR gantry, which has a 60-cm bore. Using APDs as readout electronics of the scintillation crystals, the PET detector is not sensitive to the magnetic field of the 3T MRI, which has essentially the same specifications as the Siemens Verio MRI system. With a size of $4 \times 4 \times 20$ mm^3 of the LSO crystals, the PET component of the Biograph mMR offers a spatial resolution (full width at half maximum [FWHM] X/Y/Z = 4.3/4.3/4.3 mm at r = 10 mm) similar to that of the Siemens PET/CT system, the Biograph mCT. The axial extension of the FOV of the PET is 25.8 cm and that of the MRI 50 cm. The temporal performance of APDs is slower than that of PMTs so that the PET component has no TOF capability. The coincidence window is 5.9 ns compared with 4.1 ns of that of the Biograph mCT. The smaller diameter of the PET detector and longer axial extension of the Biograph mMR in comparison to the Biograph mCT leads to a sensitivity of 15 kcps/MBq (according to the NEMA NU 2-2007 protocol[19] at r = 0 cm), which is a 45% increase compared with the Biograph mCT.[29] Delso and colleagues[29] reported a peak noise equivalent count (NEC) rate of 184 kcps at 23.1 kBq/mL. The detector cassettes are water-cooled to keep the temperature of the APDs constant. Despite the full integration of the PET system within the MRI, there were no significant distortions and no visible interferences when comprehensive tests of the MR component were performed regarding magnetic field (B0) and RF field (B1) homogeneities as well as possible interferences of the PET electronics with the MR signals.[29]

Since 2010, more than 60 Biograph mMR systems have been installed or ordered worldwide. During this period the PET hardware of the Biograph mMR was not modified. To improve MR imaging, new 4-channel coils became recently available for dedicated imaging of the breast and for special purposes, such as imaging of the carotid arteries. The breast coil can be applied for both diagnostic imaging and biopsy. A prototype of the breast coil was analyzed in detail by Aklan and colleagues.[30] They found that also during simultaneous PET imaging, the breast coil provided qualitatively good MR images, whereas global PET counts were reduced by 11%. This attenuation caused by the breast coil could be corrected using a CT-based 3-D attenuation map of the coil. Special coils for breast and carotid imaging, compatible with the Biograph mMR, are also offered by RAPID Biomedical (Rimpar, Germany). The breast coil has 16 channels and the carotid coil 6. **Fig. 1** shows images of a PET/MRI investigation performed with the breast coil of RAPID Biomedical and the Biograph mMR at the Technical University Munich.[31]

To obtain information for AC of the PET data acquired by the Biograph mMR, a Dixon sequence is performed at each bed position in 18 seconds.[32] This sequence delivers in-phase and out-phase images, from which fat and water images are calculated. The segmentation of these images results in 4 tissue classes, to which the ACs of air, lung, fat, and soft tissue are assigned.

Because the FOV of the MRI has a smaller diameter than the PET ring (50 cm vs 60 cm), the peripheral parts of the patient's arms are commonly truncated in the MR images so that the transaxial attenuation factors are erroneous.[33,34] As discussed in the articles by Eldib and

colleagues,[35] different correction methods have been suggested and are applied.[25] Recently an MR imaging–based solution of this problem was proposed for the Biograph mMR so that no further correction is needed. Blumhagen and colleagues[36] compensated inhomogeneities of the B0 field and gradient nonlinearities, which are a reason for the truncation artifact at the border of MRI FOV, by using an optimal readout gradient. In this way they were able to extend the transaxial FOV of the MR image. When the B0 Homogenization Using Gradient Enhancement (HUGE) method was applied to patient data, the mean body volume increased by 5.4% and local SUV changes of up to 30% were found compared with truncation-affected data (**Fig. 2**). It is expected that this method will be included in a future upgrade of the Biograph mMR software.

Silicon Photomultipliers–Based PET/MRI

In 2014, GE announced an integrated, simultaneous PET/MRI for whole-body imaging, the SIGNA PET/MR, and installed first research systems at Stanford University; the University of California, San Francisco; and the University of Zurich (Switzerland). Currently, GE has obtained more than 20 orders worldwide so that further PET/MRI scanners have been installed in the meantime. In this hybrid scanner, the MR compatibility was also ensured by solid-state photo detectors. This time the classic magneto-sensitive PMTs of the PET detector were replaced by SiPMs, also known as Geiger-Müller mode APDs and multipixel photon counters.

Numerous articles have reported the advantages of SiPMs over APDs[37–41]: their gain of 10^6 is similar to that of PMTs, whereas the gain of APDs is just

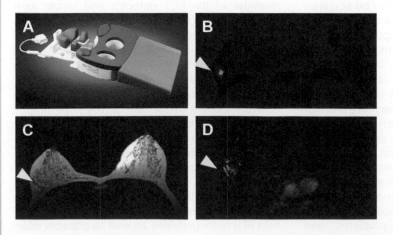

Fig. 1. PET/MR images of breast cancer performed with (*A*) a dedicated 16-channel breast coil in a Biograph mMR scanner. (*B*) The FDG uptake of the tumor (*arrow head*) is shown in the fused PET/MR image. (*C*) The lower row displays the results of a T2-weighted, turbo spin-echo sequence with fat suppression and (*D*) a subtraction image of post minus pre Gd-DTPA contrast agent injection acquired with a T1-weighted dynamic 3-D sequence. (Image courtesy of RAPID Biomedical, Germany); and *Modified from* [*B–D*] Dregely I, Lanz T, Metz S, et al. A 16-channel MR coil for simultaneous PET/MR imaging in breast cancer. Eur Radiol 2015;25(4): 1158; with permission.)

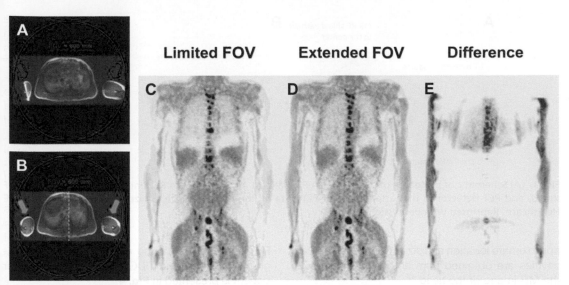

Fig. 2. Truncation correction by applying the HUGE method. (*A, B*) Transversal slice with an FOV of 600 mm. Typical distortions of the patient's arms lying at off-center positions (*A, red arrows*) were reduced using the HUGE method with an optimal readout gradient for the patient's left and right arms (*B, green arrows*). (*C*) shows the truncation artifact due to the limited FOV of the MR image, whereas (*D*) shows no truncation due to the HUGE-based extended FOV. Note that the increased transversal attenuation factor leads to an increased radiotracer uptake also in the thorax region (difference [*E*]). (*Modified from* Blumhagen JO, Braun H, Ladebeck R, et al. Field of view extension and truncation correction for MR-based human attenuation correction in simultaneous MR/PET imaging. Med Phys 2014;41:022303.)

10^2; they are faster with a rise time of approximately 300 ps compared with more than 1 ns of APDs; their supply voltage is approximately 40 V compared with approximately 400 V necessary for APDs. In several experimental studies, SiPM-equipped PET detectors – mainly designed for small animal and human brain applications – have been developed and their feasibility for PET/MRI has been tested by research groups.[42–44]

Based on the growing experience with SiPMs, GE decided to use this readout component in the PET detector of its new hybrid scanner.[45] The PET detector has a timing resolution of less than 400 ps FWHM[46] so that it has TOF capability. The scintillator crystals of sizes $4 \times 5.3 \times 25$ mm^3 are made of LYSO. Each 16×48 mm^2 block of these crystals is read out by 3×6 SiPM pixels that are mounted on a circuit board together with application-specified integrated circuits (ASICs). These ASICs provide pulse shaping, gain control, X-Y and energy determination, arrival time, trigger validation, and temperature measurements. The output signals of the ASICs are further processed on an attached digital board. Its output is transmitted over optical fibers, minimizing this way interference with the MR receiving coils.

One of the innovative features of the GE PET/MR is the so-called Compton scatter recovery, which leads to an increased system sensitivity. Events scattered within adjacent detector blocks and with energies below the discriminator energy, which are otherwise rejected, are combined, if it is concluded from their energy, position, and timing information that they belong to one 511 keV photon.

The PET detector is integrated in a modified GE Discovery 750w 3.0T MRI scanner[47] and mounted between the RF shield and the gradient coil (**Fig. 3**). To minimize attenuation of PET counts by the MR body coil, this coil and its former were redesigned. The axial FOV of the PET is 25 cm. The PET resolution is X/Y/Z = 4.2/4.2/5.7 mm (FWHM) at r = 10 mm. The sensitivity is 22.9 kcps/MBq (according to the NEMA NU 2-2007 protocol[19] at r = 0 cm) and the NEC rate is approximately 220 kps at 17 kBq/mL.[46] Both numbers decrease by less than 2% when the PET measurement was done during MR operation.

For AC, a Dixon sequence is acquired at each bed position so that fat and water images become available from which the 4 tissue classes of air, lung, fat, and soft tissue are classified.[48] As with the systems of Philips and Siemens, the MR imaging–based AC of GE does not consider bone specifically in body regions below the head. Bone is classified as soft tissue, although its linear AC is approximately 0.15 per cm compared with 0.096 per cm for soft tissue. For the head, the

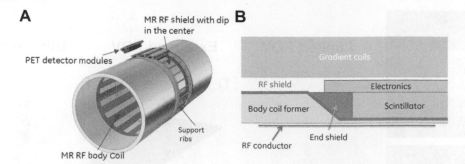

Fig. 3. (*A*) Schematic of prototype of the GE SIGNA PET/MR. (*B*) Arrangement of RF conductor of the body coil, RF shield, and PET detector so that attenuation of PET data by the body coil is minimized. (Image courtesy of GE Healthcare. Reprinted with permission.)

approximate location and size of skull bone and air cavities are obtained from an atlas registered to the MR image of the head.[47]

First clinical [18][F]-fluoro-2-deoxyglucose (FDG) images in tumor patients were presented by Iagaru and coworkers[47] and compared with images obtained with a GE Discovery 600 or 690 PET/CT scanner. When comparing such images, it has to be considered that the recording times are different with the PET/MRI acquisition, for example, 1 hour after the PET/CT study. In this period, the background of the radiotracer decreases and the uptake in the lesions may increase. A case study acquired at the University of Uppsala (Sweden) with a SIGNA

PET/MR and comparing diffusion-weighted imaging (DWI)–MRI and FDG-PET in a lung cancer patient is presented in **Fig. 4**.

A NEW PATH TO ATTENUATION CORRECTED PET IMAGES IN PET/MRI

The realization of the PET detector as a TOF-capable system, such as available with the SIGNA PET/MR and with the Ingenuity TF PET/MR, opens a new way to assess data on tissue attenuation without MR images.

Recently, previous suggestions[49,50] to determine both the attenuation map and the activity

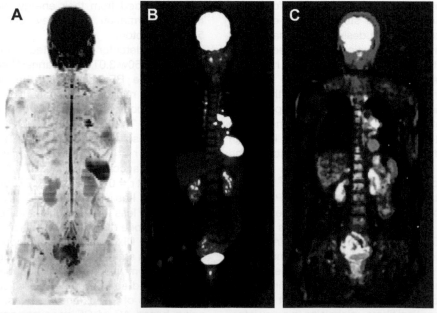

Fig. 4. PET/MR images obtained with a TOF-capable GE SIGNA PET/MR in a female lung cancer patient. (*A*) DWI–MR image and (*B*) FDG-PET image; both images present maximum intensity projections. (*C*) Fused PET/MR image showing a coronal plane. The lung tumor is displayed in both the DWI–MR image and FDG-PET image. In addition, the PET image shows uptake of FDG in brown fat along the spine. (*Courtesy of* Hakan Ahlström, MD, and Mark Lubberink, PhD, University of Uppsala, Sweden.)

distribution from emission data alone were picked up[51,52] and a new iterative reconstruction method called maximum likelihood reconstruction of attenuation and activity (MLAA)[51] was suggested. In conventional PET, this method does not lead to stable results because its solution may end in local minima, which can only be avoided by additional or prior information.[53–55] Such additional information becomes available in TOF-PET where the unknown activity to be reconstructed along an LOR is reduced by the quotient of a subject's cross-section and the width of TOF length. There are several recent articles examining the application of TOF-PET.[54–61] Currently, two of the commercial clinical PET/MR scanners offer TOF and may introduce MLAA in future software versions.

PERSPECTIVES

From the PET hardware point of view, an advance in clinical PET/MRI instrumentation can be identified from a PMT-based sequential PET/MRI system via an APD-based simultaneous PET/MRI system to a SiPM-based simultaneous PET/MRI system. In the SIGNA PET/MR, the digitization of position and energy information of the PET events is performed directly in the detector module. In this way, digital signals can be transferred to outside the PET/MRI system via optical fibers so that possible interferences with the MRI system are avoided. A further step can be achieved by solutions, such as the digital SiPM developed by Philips Digital Photon Counting (Aachen, Germany).[62–64] First reports demonstrated the feasibility of this new detector component for preclinical PET/MRI.[44,65] It may be expected that such a development will also have an impact on future clinical whole-body PET/MRI. Furthermore, a small compact and mainly digital MRI–compatible PET detector insert might be realized that can easily be installed in and removed from a standard clinical MR. Such a solution would result in a cost-efficient neuro-PET/MRI system. Beyond the advances on the PET side, MRI–related progress can be expected. The previously discussed development of the HUGE approach[36] to avoid the arm truncation serves as an example. The search for improved protocols to make PET/MRI investigations more convenient for the patient and more time efficient may lead to new MRI sequences.

SUMMARY

After the successful introduction of PET/CT, the search for appropriate PET/MRI instrumentation as another bimodal imaging tool was intensified. Research groups offered different suggestions of integrated simultaneous PET/MRI for small animal imaging. The replacement of photomultipliers by APDs as non–magneto-sensitive readout electronics of the scintillation crystals proved a promising solution. After first prototypes of a 3T PET/MRI scanner for brain imaging equipped with APDs, Siemens brought out a whole-body PET/MRI scanner at 3T using the same technology in 2010. This scanner is able to acquire PET and MRI simultaneously and is currently installed at more than 60 sites worldwide. Also in 2010, Philips installed its first sequential PET/MRI scanner with a still PMT-based, TOF-capable PET component that is linked by a common turntable to a 3T MRI scanner positioned more than 4 m away. In 2014, a first prototype of a simultaneous PET/MRI system that uses SiPMs instead of APDs as readout components was delivered by GE to 3 sites in the United States and Switzerland. Due to fast timing behavior, this PET/MRI system has TOF capability. It can be expected that SiPM-based PET detectors with additional digital signal processing at their front end represent the future PET technology of choice. Looking at the MRI component of current PET/MRI systems, primary improvements come from sequences and new coils.

ACKNOWLEDGMENTS

The authors thank Professor Syed M. Qaim (Institute of Neuroscience and Medicine – 5) for proofreading the final article.

REFERENCES

1. Pietrzyk U, Herholz K, Heiss WD. Three-dimensional alignment of functional and morphological tomograms. J Comput Assist Tomogr 1990;14:51–9.
2. Burger C, Buck A. Requirements and implementation of a flexible kinetic modeling tool. J Nucl Med 1997;38:1818–23.
3. Beyer T, Townsend DW, Brun T, et al. A combined PET/CT scanner for clinical oncology. J Nucl Med 2000;41:1369–79.
4. Townsend DW. A combined PET/CT scanner: the choices. J Nucl Med 2001;42:533–4.
5. Shao Y, Cherry SR, Farahani K, et al. Simultaneous PET and MR imaging. Phys Med Biol 1997;42:1965–70.
6. Pichler B, Lorenz E, Mirzoyan R, et al. Performance test of a LSO-APD PET module in a 9.4 tesla magnet. IEEE NSS-MIC Conference Record. Toronto, Canada, November 8–14, 1998. p. 1237–9.
7. Catana C, Wu Y, Judenhofer MS, et al. Simultaneous acquisition of multislice PET and MR images: initial

results with a MR-compatible PET scanner. J Nucl Med 2006;47:1968–76.

8. Judenhofer MS, Catana C, Swann BK, et al. PET/MRI images, acquired with a compact MRI compatible PET detector in a 7 Tesla magnet. Radiology 2007; 244:807–14.

9. Judenhofer MS, Wehrl HF, Newport DF, et al. Simultaneous PET-MRI: a new approach for functional andmorphological imaging. Nat Med 2008; 14:459–65.

10. Wehrl HF, Sauter AW, Judenhofer MS, et al. Combined PET/MRIimaging—technology and applications. Technol Cancer Res Treat 2010;9:5–20.

11. Pichler BJ, Judenhofer MS, Catana C, et al. Performance test of an LSO-APD detector in a 7-T MRI scanner for simultaneous PET/MRI. J Nucl Med 2006;47:639–47.

12. Schmand M, Burbar Z, Corbeil J, et al. BrainPET: first human tomograph for simultaneous (functional) PET and MR imaging. J Nucl Med 2007;48(Suppl 2): 310P.

13. Schlemmer HP, Pichler B, Schmand M, et al. Simultaneous MR/PET imaging of the human brain: feasibility study. Radiology 2008;248:1028–35.

14. Herzog H, Langen KJ, Weirich C, et al. High resolution BrainPET combined with simultaneous MRI. Nuklearmedizin 2011;50:74–82.

15. Kolb A, Wehrl HF, Hofmann M, et al. Technical performance evaluation of a human brain PET/MRI system. Eur Radiol 2012;22:1776–88.

16. Catana C, van der Kouwe A, Benner T, et al. Toward implementing an MRI-based PET attenuation-correction method for neurologic studies on the MR-PET brain prototype. J Nucl Med 2010;51: 1431–8.

17. Ratib O, Willi JP, Wissmeyer M, et al. Clinical application of whole body hybrid PET-MR scanner in oncology. Eur J Nucl Med Mol Imaging 2010; 37(Suppl 2):S220.

18. Surti S, Kuhn A, Werner ME, et al. Performance of Philips Gemini TF PET/CT scanner with special consideration for its time-of-flight imaging capabilities. J Nucl Med 2007;48:471–80.

19. National Electrical Manufacturers Association. NEMA standards publication NU 2–2007. Rosslyn (VA): National Electrical Manufacturers Association; 2007. Performance measurements of positron emission tomographs.

20. Zaidi H, Ojha N, Morich M, et al. Design and performance evaluation of a whole-body Ingenuity TF PET-MRI system. Phys Med Biol 2011; 56:3091–106.

21. Kalemis A, Delattre BM, Heinzer S. Sequential whole-body PET/MR scanner: concept, clinical use, and optimisation after two years in the clinic. The manufacturer's perspective. MAGMA 2013;26: 5–23.

22. Mullani NA, Markham J, Ter-Pogossian MM. Feasibility of time-of-flight reconstruction in positron emission tomography. J Nucl Med 1980;21:1095–7.

23. Budinger TF. Time-of-flight positron emission tomography: status relative to conventional PET. J Nucl Med 1983;24:73–8.

24. Herzog H, van den Hoff J. Combined PET/MR systems: an overview and comparison of currently available options. Q J Nucl Med Mol Imaging 2012;56: 247–67.

25. Izquierdo D, Catana C. Magnetic resonance imaging-guided attenuation correction of positron emission tomography data in PET/MRI. PET Clinics 2016, in press.

26. Hu Z, Ojha N, Renisch S, Schulz V, et al. MR-based attenuation correction for a whole-body sequential PET/MR system. IEEE NSS-MIC Conference Record. Orlando, FL, October 25–31, 2009. p. 3508–12.

27. Hu Z, Renisch S, Schweizer B, et al. MR-based attenuation correction for whole-body PET/MR system. IEEE NSS-MIC Conference Record. October 30 – November 6, 2010, Knoxville, TN. p. 2119–22.

28. Schulz V, Torres-Espallardo I, Renisch S, et al. Automatic, three-segment, MR-based attenuation correction for whole-body PET/MR data. Eur J Nucl Med Mol Imaging 2011;38:138–52.

29. Delso G, Fürst S, Jakoby B, et al. Performance measurements of the Siemens mMR integrated wholebody PET/MR scanner. J Nucl Med 2011;52: 1914–22.

30. Aklan B, Paulus DH, Wenkel E, et al. Toward simultaneous PET/MR breast imaging: systematic evaluation and integration of a radiofrequency breast coil. Med Phys 2013;40:024301.

31. Dregely I, Lanz T, Metz S, et al. A 16-channel MR coil for simultaneous PET/MR imaging in breast cancer. Eur Radiol 2015;25(4):1154–61.

32. Martinez-Moller A, Souvatzoglou M, Delso G, et al. Tissue classification as a potential approach for attenuation correction in whole-body PET/MRI: evaluation with PET/CT data. J Nucl Med 2009;50:520–6.

33. Delso G, Martinez-Möller A, Bundschuh RA, et al. The effect of limited MR field of view in MR/PET attenuation correction. Med Phys 2010;37:2804–12.

34. Keller SH, Holm S, Hansen AE, et al. Image artifacts from MR-based attenuation correction in clinical, whole-body PET/MRI. MAGMA 2013;26:173–81.

35. Eldib M, Bini J, Faul D. Attenuation Correction for MR Coils in Combined PET/MR Imaging: a review. PET Clinics 2016, in press.

36. Blumhagen JO, Ladebeck R, Fenchel M, et al. MR-based field-of-view extension in MR/PET: B(0) homogenization using gradient enhancement (HUGE). Magn Reson Med 2012;70:1047–57.

37. Otte AN, Barral J, Dolgoshein B, et al. A test of silicon photomultipliers as readout for PET. Nucl Instrum Methods Phys Res A 2005;545:705–15.

38. Renker D. Geiger-mode avalanche photodiodes, history, properties and problems. Nucl Instrum Methods Phys Res A 2006;567:48–56.

39. Llosa G, Belcari N, Bisogni MG, et al. Silicon photo-multipliers and SiPM matrices as photodetectors in nuclear medicine. IEEE NSS-MIC Conference Record. October 27 – November 3, 2007, Honolulu, HI. p. 3220–3.

40. Roncali E, Cherry SR. Application of silicon photo-multipliers to positron emission tomography. Ann Biomed Eng 2011;39:1358–77.

41. Zaidi H, del Guerra A. An outlook on future design of hybrid PET/MRI systems. Med Phys 2011;38: 5667–89.

42. Schaart DR, van Dam HT, Seifert S, et al. A novel, SiPM-array-based, monolithic scintillator detector for PET. Phys Med Biol 2009;54:3501–12.

43. Yoon HS, Ko GB, Kwon SI, et al. Initial results of simultaneous PET/MRI experiments with an MRI-compatible silicon photomultiplier PET scanner. J Nucl Med 2012;53:608–14.

44. Wehner J, Weissler B, Dueppenbecker PM, et al. MR-compatibility assessment of the first preclinical PET-MRI insert equipped with digital silicon photo-multipliers. Phys Med Biol 2015;60:2231–55.

45. Available at: http://www3.gehealthcare.com/en/products/categories/magnetic_resonance_imaging/signa_pet-mr#tabs/tab6C656B65BE3D48D1934AC9A8EA94E0AD. Accessed October 21, 2015.

46. Levin C, Deller T, Peterson W, et al. Initial results of simultaneous whole-body ToF PET/MR. J Nucl Med 2014;55(Suppl 1):660.

47. Iagaru A, Mittra E, Minamimoto R, et al. Simulta-neous whole-body time-of-flight 18F-FDG PET/MRI: a pilot study comparing SUVmax with PET/CT and assessment of MR image quality. Clin Nucl Med 2015;40:1–8.

48. Wollenweber SD, Ambwani S, Lonn AHR, et al. Com-parison of 4-Class and continuous Fat/Water methods for whole-body, MR-based PET attenuation correction. IEEE Trans Nucl Sci 2013;60:3391–8.

49. Censor Y, Gustafson DE, Lent A, et al. New approach to the emission computerized tomography problem: simultaneous calculation of attenuation and activity coefficients. IEEE Trans Nucl Sci 1979; 27:2775–9.

50. Natterer F, Herzog H. Attenuation correction in positron emission tomography. Math Meth Appl Sci 1992;15:321–30.

51. Nuyts J, Dupont P, Stroobants S, et al. Simultaneous maximum a posteriori reconstruction of attenuation

and activity distributions from emission sinograms. IEEE Trans Med Imaging 1999;18:393–403.

52. Glatting G, Wuchenauer M, Reske SN. Simultaneous iterative reconstruction for emission and attenuation images in positron emission tomography. Med Phys 2000;27:2065–71.

53. Natterer F. Attenuation correction in emission tomog-raphy. In: Sabatier P, editor. Inverse problems. New York: NY Academic Press; 1987. p. 21–33.

54. Defrise M, Rezaei A, Nuyts J. Transmission-less attenuation correction in time-of-flight PET: analysis of a discrete iterative algorithm. Phys Med Biol 2014;59:1073–95.

55. Mehranian A, Zaidi H. Joint estimation of activity and attenuation in whole-body TOF PET/MRI using con-strained Gaussian mixture models. IEEE Trans Med Imaging 2015;34(9):1808–21.

56. Mehranian A, Zaidi H. Impact of time-of-flight PET on quantification errors in MRI-based attenuation correction. J Nucl Med 2015;56:635–41.

57. Mehranian A, Zaidi H. Clinical assessment of emis-sion- and segmentation-based MRI-guided attenua-tion correction in whole body TOF PET/MRI. J Nucl Med 2015;56:877–83.

58. Salomon A, Goedicke A, Schweizer B, et al. Simulta-neous reconstruction of activity and attenuation for PET/MR. IEEE Trans Med Imaging 2011;30:804–13.

59. Rezaei A, Defrise M, Bal G, et al. Simultaneous reconstruction of activity and attenuationin time-of-flight PET. IEEE Trans Med Imaging 2012;31: 2224–33.

60. Defrise M, Rezaei A, Nuyts J. Time-of-flight PET data determine the attenuation sinogram up to a con-stant. Phys Med Biol 2012;57:885–99.

61. Boellaard R, Hofman M, Hoekstra O, et al. Accurate PET/MR quantification using time of flight MLAA im-age reconstruction. Mol Imag Biol 2014;16:469–77.

62. Available at: http://www.digitalphotoncounting.com/. Accessed October 21, 2015.

63. Frach T, Prescher G, Degenhardt C, et al. The digital silicon photomultiplier – system architecture and performance evaluation. IEEE NSS-MIC Conference Record. October 30 – November 6, 2010, Knoxville, TN. p. 1722–7.

64. Seifert S, van der Lei G, van Dam HT, et al. First characterization of a digital SiPM based time-of-flight PET detector with 1 mm spatial resolution. Phys Med Biol 2013;58:3061–74.

65. Schulz V, Weissler B, Gebhardt P, et al. Initial results of a preclinical simultaneous 3T PET/MR insert with new fully digital silicon photomultipliers. J Nucl Med 2013;54(Suppl 2):149.

Innovations in Small-Animal PET/MR Imaging Instrumentation

Charalampos Tsoumpas, PhD[a], Dimitris Visvikis, PhD[b],
George Loudos, PhD[c],*

KEYWORDS

- Attenuation correction • Input function • Kinetic modeling • Low dose • Motion correction
- PET/MR imaging • Silicon photomultiplier • Time of flight

KEY POINTS

- PET/MR imaging hardware is directed toward the development of dedicated animal or organ imaging systems by exploiting all recent advances in instrumentation.
- PET/MR imaging software focuses on improving the PET aspects in different areas, such as positron range; motion; attenuation; scatter; coil artifacts; input function; partial volume; low dose; anatomic priors; kinetic modeling.
- Despite the on-going debate on the clinical usefulness of the technology, PET/MR imaging remains a promising field for innovation for both hardware and software research in nuclear imaging.

INTRODUCTION: HARDWARE CHALLENGES

Over the past 15 years, the advent of multimodality imaging, initially with the development of PET/computed tomography (CT) and single-photon emission computed tomography (SPECT)/CT and more recently with the introduction of PET/MR imaging, has led to the promise of a more detailed exploration of different physiologic processes. In PET/magnetic resonance (MR), the capability of simultaneously following different, but complementary, processes could be a major advantage in disease diagnosis and therapy assessment. The history and evolution of PET/MR imaging technology have been described in many beautiful reviews.[1–3] Some key points in the evolution of PET/MR were (1) the development of a small MR-compatible PET insert with the scintillators placed inside the MR field and optical fibers driving the light to the photomultiplier tubes and electronics, which demonstrated the feasibility of the technology[4]; (2) the use of the MR-compatible avalanche photon diodes (APDs), which led to the clinical Siemens mMR device,[5] now installed in more than 40 sites worldwide; and (3) the discovery and application of silicon photomultipliers (SiPMs), which have been used by numerous groups to design full preclinical and clinical systems.[6]

The clinical usefulness of PET/MR imaging has not been as obvious as for PET/CT and the introduction of the first whole-body PET/MR imaging scanner was—and is still—received with skepticism, but prospect too.[7,8] Although the "killer" application is yet to be found, the first clinical examinations raised new questions, mostly related to image quantification and the positive or negative

Disclosure Statement: The authors have nothing to disclose.
[a] Division of Biomedical Imaging, Faculty of Medicine and Health, University of Leeds, 8.001a, Worsley Building, Clarendon Way, Leeds LS2 9JT, UK; [b] LaTIM UMR 1101, INSERM, University of Brest, Bat 1, 1er etage, 5 avenue Foch, Brest 29609, France; [c] Department of Biomedical Engineering, Technological Educational Institute of Athens, Ag. Spiridonos 28, Egaleo, Athens 12210, Greece
* Corresponding author.
E-mail address: gloudos@teiath.gr

PET Clin 11 (2016) 105–118
http://dx.doi.org/10.1016/j.cpet.2015.10.005
1556-8598/16/$ – see front matter © 2016 Elsevier Inc. All rights reserved.

effects of replacing CT with MR imaging.[9] Software research has focused on improving PET corrections either by taking advantage of the MR imaging information or by trying to predict missing CT data. In parallel, the advances in the field of MR-compatible detectors made feasible the construction and evaluation of detector modules with superior performance compared with the existing clinical PET/MR imaging. The SiPM technology is now following 2 directions, analog and digital, with the first being recently clinically adopted by GE Healthcare in the SIGNA clinical system.[10] The advantages of SiPMs are well known and have been demonstrated by many groups over the past decade. However, besides MR compatibility, SiPMs also have promising characteristics, including (1) low costs, especially when produced in large scale; (2) compact size, which allows the construction of really flexible and adoptable systems; (3) time-of-flight (TOF) capability; and (4) low power supply. All of these are likely to lead to new efficient systems in the near future.

There are numerous reviews on both technical and clinical aspects of PET/MR imaging, published during the past 5 years, which make it rather hard to avoid duplicating what is already written. However, in 2011, a pan-European network on PET/MR imaging was funded by the European Cooperation in Science and Technology (COST) Office, with the active authors' participation. This network included more than 50 groups from Europe, ranging from hardware and software to bimodal tracers and applications. Its main objective was to improve the coordination of PET/MR imaging research, at least on the European level. Some positive outcomes were the initiation of the International Series of "PSMR Conference on PET/MR imaging and SPECT/MR imaging," the organization of 2 "International Summer Schools on PET/MR Engineering," the organization of several workshops and special sessions on PET/MR, the financial support of more than 50 students who carried out part of their research in different laboratories, and the submission of many European, International, and National projects, some of which were approved and are now being implemented. Thus, in this article, the authors attempt to provide some inside information on the scientific work carried out in the field, which is currently generating more mature outcomes and subsequent research projects. In the context of this article, prototypes or systems (not separate modules), which have been developed, are under development, or have been proposed and exploit the recent advances of PET/MR instrumentation are focused on. These systems can be divided into 2 main categories: small-animal systems and dedicated clinical systems. The software challenges, which are obviously applicable to both categories, are also reviewed.

Small-animal Imaging Systems

The first reported system for small-animal imaging was developed by Pichler and colleagues[11] and used the combination of lutetium oxyorthosilicate (LSO) with APDs, which was the state-of-the-art technology at this time. The system had an outer diameter of 120 mm and was placed inside the gradient of a 7-T MR imaging scanner, while the radiofrequency (RF) coil had an outer diameter of 60 mm and inner diameter of 36 mm and fitted inside the PET ring. Each detector had 19×19 mm^2 crystal blocks, and each block consisted of a 12×12 array of $1.5 \times 1.5 \times 4.5$ mm^3 LSO crystals. Each crystal block was placed on a monolithic 3×3 APD array, with an active area of 5×5 mm^2 for each APD. The system showed very good performance with no interference from the magnetic field and reported energy resolution of $\sim$15%. All crystal pixels were clearly resolved, and successful simultaneous mouse imaging was performed.

Subsequently, in terms of the HYPERImage EU FP7 project, a simultaneous animal PET/MR insert was built, where for the first time SiPM technology was assessed.[12] The system had a 99-mm axial and 160-mm transverse field of view (FOV) and was placed inside a 3-T MR imaging scanner (Philips 3.0T, Achieve MR imaging). It consisted of 6 PET detector stacks: each one based on an array of 22×22 lutetium–yttrium oxyorthosilicate (LYSO) pixels with $10 \times 1.3 \times 1.3$ mm^3 size, mounted on a block of 64 SiPMs with a size of 4×4 mm^2 each. The signals were read by 2 dedicated 32-channel application-specific integrated circuits (ASICs), which collected energy and timing information. A signal processing unit preprocessed raw data and provided bias voltage to the SiPMs. The energy resolution was better than 11%; the timing resolution was 325 ps, and tomographic resolution was 1.6 mm.

Using similar technology, Ko and colleagues[13] developed a PET-MR insert, which was placed inside a 9.4-T Agilent MR imaging scanner. The system had a 55-mm axial FOV and included 4 rings of 16 detectors. Each detector was based on a 9×9 LYSO array with $1.2 \times 1.2 \times 10$ mm^3 pixels coupled to a 4×4 channel multipixel photon counter. The energy resolution was 12.4%; the maximum sensitivity was 3.4%, and the best transaxial spatial resolution was 0.79 mm at the center of the FOV.

The successor of the HYPERImage was the SUBLIMA project,[14] and the major evolution was the shift to digital SiPMs.[15] The system had a 46-mm axial and 100-mm transverse FOV and was placed in a

3-T MR imaging scanner. It consisted of 10 PET detector modules with 6 stacks each. Each stack had 30 × 30 crystals with a size of 12 × 1.0 × 1.0 mm^3, coupled to an 8 × 8 digital silicon photomultiliers (dSiPM) array (DPC 3200-22-44 Philips Digital Counting) and an field-programmable gate array. The energy resolution was found equal to 12.6%, and the best timing resolution was 260 ps.

This technology was exploited for the development of digiPET,[16] which was designed for rat-brain imaging and included 4 square detectors, placed at the minimum possible distance forming a square with sides of 34.5 mm, defining an FOV of 32 × 32 × 32 mm^3. Each detector consisted of a monolithic LYSO crystal of 32 × 32 × 2 mm^3, coupled to a dSiPM. The low thickness of the scintillator and the lack of pixelization allowed improved spatial resolution by using a maximum likelihood algorithm for position estimation. The energy resolution was 18%, timing resolution 680 ps, spatial resolution 0.7 mm, and count rate 6.0 cps/kBq at the center of the FOV.

The most recent development for mouse imaging, based on dSiPMs, was presented by Weissler and colleagues.[17] The system was based on the combination of dSiPMs with LYSO crystals and its FOV was 160 mm (transaxial) and 96.6 mm (axial). Each detector block had an array of 30 × 30 crystals with a size of 0.930.93 × 12 mm^3. The reported energy resolution was 12.6%; the spatial resolution was 0.73 mm^3, and the timing resolution ranged from 260 to 565 ps. Simultaneous PET/MR imaging resolved 0.8-mm rods and provided impressive mouse images in tumor and cardiac studies, including cardiac and respiratory gating, as is shown in **Fig. 1**.

Commercial Systems

Part of this technology has been adopted by industry and led to commercially available systems, although most of them in a way still balance between product and custom prototype. Ongoing research projects and existing or new collaborations between academic and industrial partners facilitate the transfer of successful technological concepts to the market. Taking into account the potential of the domain and the engineering research, which is mainly carried out by academia, new products are expected in the near future. However, a possible bottleneck that should not be ignored is the cost and complexity of the technology, which cannot allow the absorption of multiple systems, although most manufacturers now support systems upgrade.

At the moment, the most successful commercial PET/MR imaging solution is the NanoScan system

(**Fig. 2**), offered by Mediso. In its initial version,[18] the system was sequential, equipped with a 1-T permanent magnet. The axial FOV of the system was 94 mm and the maximum transaxial FOV was 120 mm. The PET detector had 12 modules and each one comprised a 39 × 41 array of 1.12 × 1.2 × 13-mm LYSO scintillators with 1.17-mm pitch. This array was coupled to a block of 2 PSPMTs, which was magnetically shielded. Evaluation with National Electrical Manufacturers Association (NEMA) standards provided a spatial resolution of 1.35 to 2.01 mm and allowed 0.8-mm rods of a Derenzo phantom to be resolved. The maximum sensitivity was measured equal to 8.41, and the maximum count rate was 406 kcps. The recent update of the system offered an axial FOV of 100 mm and a transaxial FOV of 80 mm. Timing resolution was 1.5 ns and energy resolution was 19%. The system is provided with 2 MR imaging options (3-T clinical field strength and a 7-T high field strength), based on a cryogen-free magnet with low fringe field, as a result of a recent collaboration of the company with RS2D. The adoption of SiPM technology, as it was recently announced, is expected to soon lead to a simultaneous PET/MR imaging system.[19]

In terms of a national funded project, Trifoil Imaging is developing the LabPET/MR imaging scanner.[20] The system consists of a 164-mm ring PET detector, based on the combination of LYSO/LGSO crystals coupled to APDs, which is placed in front of a 3-T superconducting magnet. The LabPET component is based on the phoswich concept of side-to-side scintillator crystals with pixel size of 2 × 2 × 12 mm^3 for LYSO and 2 × 2 × 14 mm^3 for LGSO, each one coupled to an APD with dimensions 1.8 × 4.4 mm^2.[21] The transaxial FOV is 100 mm, and axial can vary from 37.4 to 114 mm depending on the number of rings. The energy resolution is ~25% for both scintillators; the best spatial resolution is 1.51 mm, and the sensitivity can reach 4.3% for the 11.4-cm FOV, while the highest count rate can reach 362 kcps. With the magnetic field on and the use of maximum likelihood expectation maximization, no distortions are noticeable, and the system spatial resolution is found at ~0.96 mm, while successful sequential MR and PET mouse brain and gate cardiac images were obtained.

A truly simultaneous option is the MRS (MR spectroscopy)-PET, which is offered by MR Solutions and relies on the SiPM technology, as well as the exploitation of a dual layer LYSO matrix, with pixels having $\frac{1}{2}$-pixel offset for extraction of depth of interaction information. The transaxial FOV is 70 mm, while the axial FOV depends on

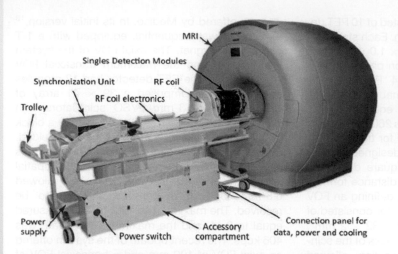

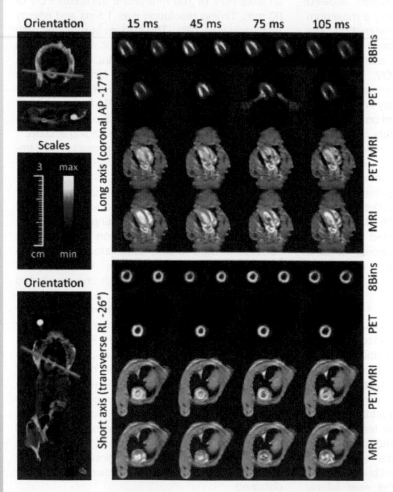

Fig. 1. (*top*) The PET/RF insert "Hyperion II^D" mounted on the patient table of a clinical 3-T MR imaging system. (*bottom*) Dual-gated (respiratory and ECG [electrocardiogram]) simultaneous PET/MR measurement of a mouse heart. Indicative slices at different time bins. (*From* Weissler B, Gebhardt P, Duppenbecker P, et al. A digital preclinical PET/MRI insert and initial results. IEEE Trans Med Imaging 2015;34(11):2258–70; with permission.)

the number of rings and varies between 45 mm for 1 ring up to 135 mm for 3 rings. Using ordered subset expectation maximization (OSEM), the best spatial resolution was found equal to 0.9 mm. Currently, only these performance indicators are given through the manufacturer's Web site.[22]

Very recently, Cubresa announced in the PSRM 2015 Conference its PET/MR imaging solution, which includes a PET insert compatible with a 7-T magnet. Two options are given: the first has a 50-mm transaxial and 66-mm axial FOV and the second has a 50-mm transaxial and 99-mm axial FOV,

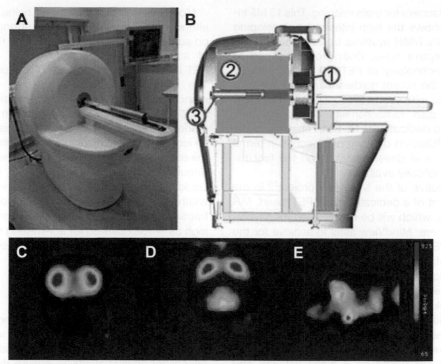

Fig. 2. (*A*) Nanoscan small-animal PET/MR scanner and (*B*) its schematics, showing the PET ring (1), magnet (2), and RF coil (3). Fused 3D MR (fast spin echo) and PET images of striatum (*C, D*) and hypophysis (*E*) using ^{11}C-FLB457 (summation image, 5–60 min after injection) of healthy male Wistar rat. (This research was originally published in *JNM*. Nagy K, Tóth M, Major P, et al. Performance evaluation of the small-animal nanoscan PET/MRI system. J Nucl Med 2013;54(10):1825–32. © by the Society of Nuclear Medicine and Molecular Imaging, Inc.)

respectively. Simultaneous images from mouse cardiac images were presented, but no additional technical details of the system were given.

Dedicated Clinical Systems

The increased acceptance of mMR, the positive feedback from the sequential Ingenuity TF PET/MR provided by Philips as well as the trimodality PET/CT MR offered by General Electric Healthcare highlighted potential clinical applications of this technology.[2] The drawbacks that this first generation had due to lack of simultaneous information or because of performance limitations encouraged several groups to propose dedicated inserts for clinical application. These concepts attracted remarkable resources from funding agencies, supporting the potential clinical impact of PET/MR if advanced systems become available.

The first whole-body clinical system that exploited SiPM technology and provided TOF capability was the SIGNA PET/MR manufactured by GE.[23] The PET insert was centered inside the MR gradient set of a GE MR 750-W 3-T scanner. It had 5 rings of 112 detector blocks with 25-cm axial and 60-cm transaxial FOV. Each block was composed of a 4 × 9 array of LYSO crystals with

$3.95 \times 5.3 \times 25 \text{ mm}^3$, coupled to a 1×3 SiPM array. The performance of this system was summarized by an energy resolution of 10.5%, timing resolution of 399 ps, transaxial spatial resolution of 3.9 mm at 1 cm from the isocenter, and a NEMA sensitivity of ~23.5 cps/kBq.[24]

Hong and colleagues[25] developed a ring brain PET, with 12.9-mm axial and 250-mm transaxial FOV. The insert consisted of 72 detector modules placed inside a 3-T MR imaging scanner. Each PET module was based on a 4 × 4 LYSO array with $3 \times 3 \times 20 \text{ mm}^3$ crystal pixels, coupled to a 4×4 SiPM array with $2.85 \times 2.85 \text{ mm}^2$ pixel size. The signals were transferred to the preamplification boards using 3-m-long flat cables, with all electronics positioned outside the MR bore. The average energy resolution was 18%, the timing resolution 4.23 ns, the best spatial resolution 3.1 mm, and the sensitivity 0.33% at the center of the FOV, with no significant effect during simultaneous MR.

Ongoing Hardware Developments

In 2013 and in terms of the 7th Framework Program, the European Union funded 2 similar projects, which aimed at the development of

PET/MR scanners for brain imaging. This 13 M$ investment shows the high interest for developing dedicated PET/MR systems besides the existing general purpose ones. Both projects aimed to push the technology of PET/MR to its limits by integrating the recent hardware and software developments, with the active cooperation of clinicians but also radiochemists developing new radiotracers dedicated to PET/MR imaging. However, they followed different approaches in terms of technological developments, and the first results are publically available.

The objective of the MindView project[26] is the development of a dedicated brain PET insert, MR compatible, which will be mainly used for psychiatric disorders. MindView aims to achieve for the first time PET resolution of ~1 mm. According to the work plan, the PET will be mounted together with a birdcage-type repetition time (TR) RF coil, and the effective aperture will be 27 cm. Each detector block will be based on large 12 × 12 SiPM arrays; different LYSO crystal configurations are currently tested to optimize performance in terms of spatial resolution and sensitivity. The readout electronics are based on a diode network and reduce the collected SiPMs signals before amplification, digitization, and position calculation. Recent results have shown that it is possible to resolve $1.5 \times 1.5 \times 10$ mm^3 crystals and achieve energy resolution of 10%, while 2-cm monolithic crystals have been tested, providing a uniform spatial resolution of 1.5 mm in 3 dimensions (3D).

On the other hand, TRIMAGE represents the first effort toward the development of a full PET/MR system.[27] The consortium develops a 1.5-T compact brain optimized MR scanner, which is designed to be compatible, from the beginning, with the PET insert that has 31-cm axial FOV. The PET component consists of 216 modules of 2.5×2.5 cm^2, arranged in 18 rectangular detectors of 5×15 cm^2, the latter in the axial direction to form a full ring of 31 cm diameter. Each module consists of a dual-layer LYSO matrix read out by 2 arrays of 4×8 SiPMs and an ASIC. The envisaged performance of the system is 2-mm spatial resolution and ~10% sensitivity.

More dedicated systems are being proposed, although their construction will strongly depend on successful funding. Very recently, the concept of a high-resolution, ultralow-dose multimodal PET insert for pediatric imaging was presented.[28] The proposed design exploits the well-tested monolithic scintillators and consists of a $32 \times 32 \times 22$ mm^3 LYSO crystal with dual-sided readout using dSiPM arrays. The design targets an isotropic spatial resolution of less than 2 mm in the entire FOV and less than 150 ps time resolution. Simulated studies have shown that the system could achieve a spatial resolution of ~2.0 mm full width at half maximum in each direction, a scatter fraction of ~32%, and a line source sensitivity as high as ~188 cps/kBq for a 1-m-long scanner.

In **Fig. 3**, the concepts of the 3 systems are shown.

SOFTWARE CHALLENGES

There are numerous software challenges associated with high-resolution, accurate, and precise PET-MR imaging.[29] On the one hand, there are necessary developments to ensure the quantitative accuracy of the reconstructed images. On the other hand, synergistic approaches can exploit the simultaneously acquired information in order to improve overall image quality. These goals can be achieved by integrating all existing aspects, such as novel TOF capabilities,[30] point-spread-function modeling,[31] physiologic motion compensation,[32] within a fast regularized list-mode[33] reconstruction using anatomic priors[34]; this includes correction for the effects of photon attenuation[35,36] and scatter[37,38] using transmission sources or appropriately preprocessed MR images. Attenuation artifacts from MR coils,[39] for example, for imaging the carotid arteries,[40] require special handling because they may cause inconsistencies in the reconstruction, thus producing image artifacts. Although attenuation and scatter can be difficult to correct, the availability of TOF has been shown to minimize the artifacts due to the improved consistency and provide an estimate of the attenuation probability map.[41] Clearly, the

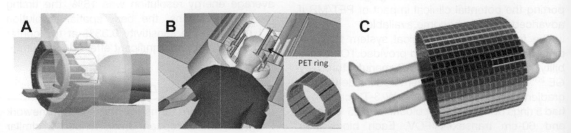

Fig. 3. Concept of the (*A*) mindview project, (*B*) trimage project, and (*C*) pediatric PET. (*Data from* Refs.[26–28])

simultaneous acquisition of PET and MR data sets represents a substantial advantage in patient physiologic motion management strategies. The effects of respiratory[42] and bulk motion[43] create image resolution degradation, which substantially reduces the ability of detection of small functional abnormalities as well as quantitative accuracy, which is essential for therapy response monitoring. In particular, for the detection of small metastases, tone must achieve at least 3-mm resolution; therefore, motion detection and correction of less than 3 mm accuracy are necessary, as some lesions may not have particularly high radiotracer uptake.[44] Furthermore, it has been shown that positron range, particularly for ^{68}Ga and ^{82}Rb radiotracers,[45] can have tremendous nonisotropic resolution degradation effects. Therefore, special care is needed to model positron range effects in the reconstruction.[46] Physiologic motion may also result in alterations in intratumor activity distribution, which in turn leads to potential errors in PET image-derived parameters characterizing tumor heterogeneity, which were recently shown as independent predictive and prognostic factors in cancer management.[47] Additional modeling of the partial volume effects[48] using information from MR either after reconstruction[49,50] or during PET image reconstruction[51] represents one of the potential advantages of PET-MR systems. Finally, the fact that the PET data acquisition is not the limiting factor in terms of overall PET/MR study duration (MR imaging requires substantially longer acquisition times than CT) offers 2 separate capabilities: (1) exploration of dynamic PET imaging,[52] and (2) lower-dose injection protocols without compromise of overall image quality.[53] Finally, the availability of simultaneous PET and MR data can allow joint PET-MR kinetic modeling techniques, which may offer an improved accuracy in the estimation of different physiologic parameters.[54]

Magnetic Resonance-based Motion Estimation

MR has much higher capabilities with respect to spatiotemporal resolution compared with PET; thus, it can be used to derive motion information, which can be subsequently used to correct for motion either after reconstruction or during the PET reconstruction process. There are different approaches for motion estimation with MR that have demonstrated utility for PET motion correction either in brain studies[55] or in the torso.[56] One of the most advanced approaches is the combination of motion measurement sequences with motion modeling. The motion measurement is

necessary for the computation of the motion fields according to the respiratory position. For example, a T1-weighted TFE (turbo field echo) sequence (TR/TE [echo time] = 3.3 ms/0.9 ms, flip angle of 10°) with parallel imaging (sensitivity encoding) applied in both phase-encoding directions allows the acquisition of the whole-thorax volume (FOV: 500 × 450 × 245 mm^3) with a spatial resolution of 1.5 × 4.1 × 5 mm^3 (feet-head, right-left, anterior-posterior).[57] However, the MR technique should not be used only for motion estimation. For that purpose, the 4-dimensional (4D) sequence is applied only at the start of the scan and then during the normal PET scan only a navigator signal is acquired for gating purposes. The MR signal can be acquired with or without navigators, and data can be sorted accordingly to enhance accuracy of motion estimation.[58]

Within the context of motion modeling, the use of generic motion models has been also proposed. The objective is the creation of a global respiratory motion model based on principal component analysis using multiple 4D T1 MR imaging patient studies covering the thoracic region. This model can then be adapted on a specific patient using only 2 breath-hold 3D MR imaging volumes in addition to 2-dimensional image navigators acquired throughout the PET/MR acquisition.[59]

The 4D images are used to estimate motion vectors with image registration techniques[60] and the navigator signal to characterize the position of the patient during the scan. Advanced motion modeling techniques can be used to estimate respiratory motion throughout the PET-MR scan.[61] These techniques are limited to the MR-based information, which does not hold details within regions that are particularly important for PET imaging, such as lungs and bone. Special sequences need to be created for capture of motion within the lungs and the bone. The latter is particularly important for accurate 4D attenuation and scatter compensation.[62]

An alternative involves the use of accelerated MR acquisitions, which greatly reduce the time spent on MR acquisitions for PET motion correction purposes. Such approaches can be based either on the use of compressed sensing[63] or on combined MR data and 4D deformation matrices estimation through a generalized reconstruction approach[64] and allow the determination of motion deformations based on ~60- to 90-second MR acquisitions.

Estimation of respiratory and cardiac motion of anesthetized animals is not a simple task because the respiration and cardiac cycles are very fast and the existing MR sequences cannot efficiently cope. Therefore, at the moment, most sequences include gating. One additional burden particularly for PET inserts with respect to motion estimation for PET-MR motion correction is the assurance of continuous temporal alignment, that is, synchronization of the PET clock with the MR clock. One solution has been recently suggested using a purpose-built design by detection of switching gradients.[65] Validation of motion estimation algorithms experimentally requires development of novel design of PET-MR phantoms that can perform realistic continuous nonrigid motion.[66,67]

Motion Compensated Image Reconstruction

Although it is generally expected that integration of motion information within reconstruction would improve image quality, Polycarpou and colleagues[68] demonstrated that this might not be the case due to the nonlinearity of OSEM. To this extent, Tsoumpas and colleagues[69] showed that regularization will be necessary to achieve the maximum for motion-incorporated reconstruction with respect to both image quality and quantification. Currently, only the median root prior (MRP) was investigated, but independently, Chun and Fessler[70] also showed improved results with quadratic prior for the penalized least-squares problem.

Fig. 4 shows the image improvement using motion information within regularized (with MRP) reconstruction. This algorithm has been implemented in STIR (Software for Tomographic Image Reconstruction,[71] release 2.4: http://stir.sf.net); it is freely available to the community.

Incorporation of motion compensation within a 4D reconstruction has shown superior results in comparison to the use of MR displacement fields for after reconstruction correction of respiratory synchronized PET images.[72,73] One of the potential issues, which is however not specific to the 4D reconstruction process, is the practical difficulty of addressing 4D attenuation and scatter corrections given the fact that an accurate MR-based estimation of the attenuation map for the torso is not available. Further research and development within the joint PET-MR field will be required toward this direction before the advances of 4D reconstruction will become apparent.[74]

Attenuation and Scatter Correction

Quantitative PET/MR imaging is clearly dependent on the accuracy of the PET attenuation correction. In addition, the precision of the attenuation maps can have a substantial influence on the accuracy of the scatter correction. Several different approaches are already proposed for attenuation correction in PET/MR, although most of them represent a compromise between a practical clinical implementation and associated accuracy.[36] More details are given in another article of this special issue.[75] State of the art in clinical PET/MR involves the use of standard Dixon protocols, which allow segmentation into 3 different tissues

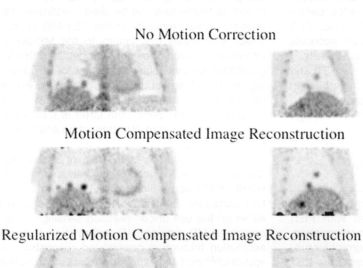

No Motion Correction

Motion Compensated Image Reconstruction

Regularized Motion Compensated Image Reconstruction

Fig. 4. Coronal and sagittal planes of reconstructed phantom demonstrating the effects due to motion (*top row*); motion correction within reconstruction (*middle row*); and motion correction within regularized MRP reconstruction (*bottom row*). Coronal and sagittal planes through different lesions of images reconstructed with 10 iterations (23 subsets). All images (displayed in SUV [standard uptake value] scale from 0 to 5) were reconstructed from simulated gated projection data (8 gates) with 50×10^6 total counts according to the simulation setup described by Tsoumpas and colleagues.[69] The images of the first 2 rows were filtered with a 6-mm isotropic 3D Gaussian kernel, whereas the image of the last row was reconstructed with penalization factor set to 400. (*Data from* Tsoumpas C, Polycarpou I, Thielemans K, et al. The effect of regularization in motion compensated PET image reconstruction: a realistic numerical 4D simulation study. Phys Med Biol 2013;58:1759–73.)

classes (air, soft tissue, fat) with fixed linear attenuation coefficient (LAC) values. The issue of this approach is the lack of consideration for bone structures, which can clearly introduce biases in the quantification of brain imaging but also for oncology applications with larger effects noted for bone lesions (up to 30% in comparison to the PET/CT derived values).[76–80] One potential solution to the bone structure identification involves the use of ultrashort echo (UTE) time sequences, as the transverse relaxation rate in bone is higher than tissue.[76] Thus, in principle, the combination of Dixon and UTE sequences can allow whole-body region classification as bone, soft tissue, fat, or air. Although UTE sequences have shown promising results in generating reasonable pseudo-CT images, difficulties remain in the accuracy of segmentation as well as the use of fixed LAC values. In addition, acquiring UTE sequences of the torso is prohibitively long to obtain a reasonable image of different parts of the body.[81] Potential solutions to the use of fixed LACs are based on the use of models relating MR intensities to CT-derived electronic densities.[82] These approaches can be combined with atlas-based solutions, aiming at exploring a database of paired CT and MR patient images. These images in combination with the acquired MR images from a given patient can then be used to derive a patient-specific pseudo-CT map.[83,84] One recent investigation by Ladefoged and colleagues[85] at the 2015 PSMR conference demonstrated that voxel-wise intensity mapping can produce brain attenuation maps with sufficient accuracy.

An attractive alternative is the estimation of the attenuation map from the PET data itself by using additional information (eg, TOF PET reconstruction[86,87]), the use of transmission information by incorporating external radioactive sources,[88,89] or even the background activity originating from the LSO crystals.[90]

Another issue concerns the need to account for the presence of MR coils and particularly their metallic components. Identifying the location of the metallic regions, which cause strong attenuation, is another challenging task. One promising methodology is the use of precalculated attenuation maps coregistered with the corresponding MR-based attenuation map.[39] The correction of the attenuation effects of coils in PET-MR is discussed in detail in another article of this special issue.[40] In addition, scatter correction can create artifacts due to the inaccuracies of the attenuation map because the single-scatter simulation strongly depends on this[91] and the smaller FOV, which would complicate the standard scaling step of the scatter estimates.[92]

Using MR for attenuation correction and scatter correction for preclinical imaging is not straightforward. For example, the automatic segmentation, which usually follows the Dixon protocol, sometimes fails when performed in animals, for example, rabbit models. On the other hand, one may think that attenuation and scatter correction, particularly in mice, are not necessary because the probability of scattering and attenuation is very small compared with larger animals or humans.[93] However, as Prasad and Zaidi[94] showed, the scatter fraction can be considerably large because of the low limit of discrimination comparing the preclinical protocols (eg, 250 keV) with the clinical protocols (eg, 450 keV). Furthermore, in PET-MR imaging, the coils will have additional attenuation and scattering effects that need to be considered appropriately.[39]

Positron Range Effects

Positron range significantly affects the imaging resolution of the PET systems, particularly for preclinical imaging.[95] When imaging inside a magnetic field, there is reduction of the positron range in perpendicular directions to the magnetic field,[96] whereas there is no variation in the direction of the magnetic field. This effect is particularly substantial for high-energy emitters, such as ^{82}Rb and ^{68}Ga, and positron range is affected by the surrounding material electron density as well as the intensity of the magnetic field.[90] Although the overall imaging resolution is improved within the magnetic field, the positron range is not reduced for magnetic fields higher than 3 T.[45] Nevertheless, there can be noticeable distortions caused by the nonisotropic resolution.[92] For example, a spherical lesion may appear ellipsoidal. To minimize this effect, Shah and colleagues[97], Kraus and colleagues[98] and Bertolli and colleagues[99] independently developed a method to reconstruct images by incorporating positron range kernels, which allows obtaining sharper images. If dedicated reconstruction is not considered, PET-MR images may suffer from positron-range artifacts in areas where low-electron-density media are present: neck and head, sinuses, and lungs. Particularly in preclinical PET imaging, development of positron range modeling approaches is indispensable.[46]

Partial Volume Effect

In brain imaging, the main effect for limiting PET resolution is partial volume with activity spilling in and out. For example, Fung and Carson[100] attempted to minimize this complication by selecting only a center line. In order to correct for partial volume, several approaches have been proposed using MR imaging. These approaches originated

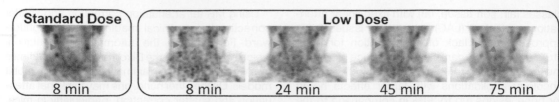

Fig. 5. Coronal PET images in the same subject using the clinical standard dose of 18F-FDG acquired for 8 minutes compared with the low-dose images acquired for 8, 25, 45, and 75 minutes. Arrows show the increased uptake in the carotids. (*Courtesy of* M. Eldib, New York, NY.)

from separate PET and MR acquisitions and have shown substantial resolution improvement.[50,101] With availability of simultaneous PET-MR systems, it is anticipated that these techniques will be translated in whole-body clinical PET-MR protocols and will help in the successful diagnosis of even smaller lesions. However, for parts of the body where motion is significant, partial volume effects can be accurately accounted for only if the motion is corrected for.[102] Partial volume correction for preclinical imaging is more imperative but it had been more challenging to ensure accurate coregistration in the past. The availability of PET inserts will enable the translation of these techniques in modeling and reconstruction of preclinical imaging techniques.

Anatomic priors
The use of MR anatomic priors within reconstruction is another plausible methodology for improving PET resolution. This idea has been proposed since the early 1990s,[103–105] primarily for brain imaging. Because of the lack of simultaneous PET-MR data, it was extremely complicated to translate the methodology in clinical practice. Once registration of PET and MR data is warranted, the second issue is the lack of coherence between function and structure.[103] For example, Vunckx and colleagues[106] evaluated a modified Bowsher algorithm[107] using nonsegmented MR images for brain PET images, and Karaoglanis and colleagues[108] studied the modified MRP[109] for imaging the myocardium. More recently, Loeb and colleagues[110] demonstrated a new approach for parametric reconstruction using Gaussian mixture models driven from anatomic MR images.

Low-dose imaging
One advantage of hybrid simultaneous PET-MR is the lack of CT. By removing CT, the opportunities for substantial dose reduction in PET increase. For example, PET acquisition can take as long as MR imaging; thus, it is reasonable to expect that new PET-MR protocols will use a substantially lower dose. A recent investigation by Eldib and colleagues[53] has shown that a substantial reduction can be achieved, as illustrated in **Fig. 5**.

Arterial Input Function and Joint Kinetic Modeling

An additional advantage for longer PET acquisitions is the plausibility of exploring dynamic imaging. The availability of the MR data sets allows segmentation of the blood pool, which can be used for the estimation of the arterial input function. The input function, for example, from carotid arteries[100] or the aorta, can offer such information: one of the difficult aspects is to locate the region of interest with relevant information, for example, carotid arteries. A recent investigation by Iguchi and colleagues[111] is another example to estimate the input function from MR. However, in torso imaging, this might be more complicated because of the effect of nonrigid motion.[112]

Very little research has focused on joint physiologic modeling from PET and MR. There is potential to extract specific physiologic biomarkers by acquiring kinetic data, using, for example, radiolabeled nanoparticles.[113] The joint analysis of kinetic data is particularly challenging, requiring accurate quantification and good temporal resolution, with no single modality providing error-free solutions. Dynamic MR imaging protocols with high temporal and spatial resolution can prove useful. Then, combined modeling of all measured data sets can provide physiologic information with potentially better accuracy and precision.

ACKNOWLEDGMENTS

The authors acknowledge the COST Action TD1007. Dr C. Tsoumpas is thankful for receiving the Leeds Mobility Award from the University of Leeds.

REFERENCES

1. Zaidi H, Del Guerra A. An outlook on future design of hybrid PET/MRI systems. Med Phys 2011; 38(10):5667–89.

2. Wehrl HF, Sauter AW, Divine MR, et al. Combined PET/MR: a technology becomes mature. J Nucl Med 2015;56(2):165–8.

3. Boellaard R, Quick HH. Current image acquisition options in PET/MR. Semin Nucl Med 2015;45(3): 192–200.

4. Raylman RR, Majewski S, Lemieux SK, et al. Simultaneous MRI and PET imaging of a rat brain. Phys Med Biol 2006;51:6371.

5. Delso G, Fürst S, Jakoby B, et al. Performance measurements of the Siemens mMR integrated whole-body PET/MR scanner. J Nucl Med 2011; 52(12):1914–22.

6. Buzhan P, Dolgoshein B, Filatov L, et al. Silicon photomultiplier and its possible applications. Nucl Instrum Methods Phys Res A 2003;504(1–3):48–52.

7. Bailey DL, Antoch G, Bartenstein P, et al. Combined PET/MR: the real work has just started. Summary report of the Third International Workshop on PET/MR Imaging; February 17–21, 2014, Tübingen, Germany. Mol Imaging Biol 2015;17(3):297–312.

8. Zaidi H, Mawlawi O. Simultaneous PET/NMR will replace PET/CT as the molecular multimodality imaging platform of choice. Med Phys 2007;34(5):1525–8.

9. Vandenberghe S, Marsden PK. PET-MRI: a review of challenges and solutions in the development of integrated multimodality imaging. Phys Med Biol 2015;60:R115.

10. Iagaru A, Minamimoto R, Levin C, et al. The potential of TOF PET-MRI for reducing artifacts in PET images. Eur J Nuc Med Mol Imag Phys 2015;2(1):A77.

11. Pichler BJ, Judenhofer MS, Catana C, et al. Performance test of an LSO-APD detector in a 7-T MRI scanner for simultaneous PET/MRI. J Nucl Med 2006;47:639–47.

12. Schulz V, Solf T, Weissler B, et al. A preclinical PET/MR insert for a human 3T MR scanner. IEEE Nuclear Science Symposium Conference Record (NSS/MIC). October 24 – November 1, 2009. p. 2577–9.

13. Ko GB, Yoon HS, Kwon SI, et al. New high performance SiPM PET insert to 9.4-T MR scanner for simultaneous PET/MRI studies. J Nucl Med 2013; 54(2):46.

14. Vandenberghe S, Thoen H, Keereman V, et al. Optimization and development of high performance TOF PET-MR systems: the SUBLIMA project. PSMR 2012 Book of Abstracts, May 2012. p. 33–4.

15. Mandai S, Charbon E. A 4 × 4 × 416 digital SiPM array with 192 TDCs for multiple high-resolution timestamp acquisition. J Inst 2013;8:P05024.

16. Espana S, Marcinkowski R, Keereman V, et al. DigiPET: sub-millimeter spatial resolution small-animal PET imaging using thin monolithic scintillators. Phys Med Biol 2014;59:3405.

17. Weissler B, Gebhardt P, Duppenbecker P, et al. A digital preclinical PET/MRI insert and initial results. IEEE Trans Med Imaging 2015;34(11): 2258–70.

18. Nagy K, Tóth1 M, Major P, et al. Performance evaluation of the small-animal nanoScan PET/MRI system. J Nucl Med 2013;54(10):1825–32.

19. Available at: http://www.mediso.com/uploaded/ NPM_3T_0615.pdf. Accessed November 2015.

20. Bricq S, Kidane HL, Lalande A, et al. Multi-modal image fusion for small animal studies in in-line PET/3T MRI. Dourdan (France): Actes des Journees RITS 201; 2015.

21. Bergeron M, Cadorette J, Tetrault MA, et al. Imaging performance of LabPET APD-based digital PET scanners for pre-clinical research. Phys Med Biol 2014;59(3):661–78.

22. Available at: http://www.mrsolutions.com/products/ imaging-systems/petmr. Accessed November 2015.

23. Delso G, Khalighi M, Hofbauer M, et al. Preliminary evaluation of image quality in a new clinical ToF-PET/MR scanner. Eur J Nuc Med Mol Imag Phys 2014;1(1):A41.

24. Levin C, Glover G, Deller T, et al. Prototype time-of-flight PET ring integrated with a 3T MRI system for simultaneous whole-body PET/MR imaging. J Nucl Med 2013;54(2):148.

25. Hong KJ, Choi Y, Jung JH, et al. A prototype MR insertable brain PET using tileable GAPD arrays. Med Phys 2013;40:042503.

26. González AJ, Majewski S, Conde P, et al. Progress report on the MindView brain PET detector module based on large area SiPMs arrays. Eur J Nuc Med Mol Imag Phys 2014;1(1):A66.

27. Del Guerra A. TRIMAGE—development of a simultaneous trimodal (PET/MR/EEG) imaging tool for early diagnosis of schizophrenia and other mental disorders. Eur Psych 2015;30(1):161.

28. Mikhaylova E, Tabacchini V, Borghi G, et al. Geometric optimization of an ultralow-dose high-resolution pediatric PET scanner based on monolithic scintillators with dSiPM readout. Eur J Nuc Med Mol Imag Phys 2015;2(1):A23.

29. Tsoumpas C, Gaitanis A. Modeling and simulation of 4D PET-CT and PET-MR images. PET Clin 2013;8(1):95–110.

30. Conti M. Why is TOF PET reconstruction a more robust method in the presence of inconsistent data? Phys Med Biol 2011;56(1):155–68.

31. Pratx G, Levin CS. Online detector response calculations for high-resolution PET image reconstruction. Phys Med Biol 2011;56:1563–84.

32. Dutta J, Huang C, Li Q, et al. Pulmonary imaging using respiratory motion compensated simultaneous PET/MR. Med Phys 2015;42:4227–40.

33. Pratx G, Surti S, Levin C. Fast list-mode reconstruction for time-of-flight PET using graphics hardware. IEEE Trans Nucl Sci 2011;58(1): 105–9.

34. Vunckx K, Atre A, Baete K, et al. Evaluation of three MRI-based anatomical priors for quantitative PET brain imaging. IEEE Trans Med Imaging 2012;31: 599–612.

35. Mehranian A, Zaidi H. Emission-based estimation of lung attenuation coefficients for PET/MR attenuation correction. Phys Med Biol 2015;60:4813.

36. Visvikis D, Monnier F, Bert J, et al. PET/MR attenuation correction: where do we come from and where are we going. Eur J Nucl Med Mol Imaging 2014;41(6):1172–5.

37. Polycarpou I, Thielemans K, Manjeshwar R, et al. Comparative evaluation of scatter correction in 3D PET using different scatter-level approximations. Ann Nucl Med 2011;25(9):643–9.

38. Gaens M, Bert J, Pietrzyk U, et al. GPU-accelerated Monte Carlo based scatter correction in brain PET/MR. IEEE Nuclear Science Symposium and Medical Imaging Conference (NSS/MIC). October 27 – November 2, 2013.

39. Eldib M, Bini J, Robson PM, et al. Markerless attenuation correction for carotid MRI surface receiver coils in combined PET/MR imaging. Phys Med Biol 2015;60:4705–17.

40. Eldib M, Bini J, Faul DD, et al. Attenuation correction for MR coils in combined PET/MR imaging. PET Clin, in press.

41. Mehranian A, Zaidi H. Joint estimation of activity and attenuation in whole-body TOF PET/MRI using constrained Gaussian mixture models. IEEE Trans Med Imaging 2015;34(9):1808–21.

42. Dikaios N, Izquierdo-Garcia D, Graves MJ, et al. MRI-based motion correction of thoracic PET: initial comparison of acquisition protocols and correction strategies suitable for simultaneous PET/MRI systems. Eur Radiol 2012;22:439–46.

43. Kolbitsch C, Prieto C, Tsoumpas C, et al. A 3D MR-acquisition scheme for non-rigid bulk motion correction in simultaneous PET-MR. Med Phys 2014;41(8):082304.

44. Polycarpou I, Tsoumpas C, King AP, et al. Impact of respiratory motion correction and spatial resolution on lesion detection in PET: a simulation study based on real MR dynamic data. Phys Med Biol 2014;59(3):697–713.

45. Eleftheriou A, Tsoumpas C, Bertolli O, et al. Effect of the magnetic field on positron range using GATE for PET-MR. Eur J Nuc Med Mol Imag Phys 2014;1:A50.

46. Cal-Gonzalez J, Perez-Liva M, Lopez-Herraiz J, et al. Tissue-dependent and spatially-variant positron range correction in 3D PET. IEEE Trans Med Imaging 2015;34(11):2394–403.

47. Hatt M, Majdoub M, Vallières M, et al. ^{18}F-FDG PET uptake characterization through texture analysis: investigating the complementary nature of heterogeneity and functional tumor volume in a multi-cancer site patient cohort. J Nucl Med 2015;56: 38–44.

48. Erlandsson K, Buvat I, Pretorius H, et al. A review of partial volume correction techniques for emission tomography and their applications in neurology, cardiology and oncology. Phys Med Biol 2012;57: R119.

49. Shidahara M, Tsoumpas C, McGinnity CJ, et al. Wavelet-based resolution recovery using an anatomical prior provides quantitative recovery for human population phantom PET [^{11}C]raclopride data. Phys Med Biol 2012;57:3107–22.

50. Le Pogam A, Hatt M, Descourt P, et al. Evaluation of a 3D local multi-resolution algorithm for the correction of partial volume effects in positron emission tomography. Med Phys 2011;38(9):4920–33.

51. Kotasidis FA, Angelis GI, Anton-Rodriguez J, et al. Isotope specific resolution recovery image reconstruction in high resolution PET imaging. Med Phys 2014;41(5):052503.

52. Wehrl HF, Hossain M, Lankes K, et al. Simultaneous PET-MRI reveals brain function in activated and resting state on metabolic, hemodynamic and multiple temporal scales. Nat Med 2015;19:1184–9.

53. Eldib M, Bini J, Lairez O, et al. Feasibility of ^{18}F-Fluorodeoxyglucose radiotracer dose reduction in simultaneous carotid PET/MR imaging. Am J Nucl Med Mol Imaging 2015;5(4):401–7.

54. Tang J, Kuwabara H, Wong DF, et al. Direct 4D reconstruction of parametric images incorporating anato-functional joint entropy. Phys Med Biol 2010;55(15):4261–72.

55. Catana C, Benner T, Van der Kouwe A, et al. MRI-assisted PET motion correction for neurologic studies in an integrated MR-PET scanner. J Nucl Med 2011;52:154–61.

56. Guerin B, Cho S, Chun SY, et al. Nonrigid PET motion compensation in the lower abdomen using simultaneous tagged-MRI and PET imaging. Med Phys 2011;38(6):3025–38.

57. Tsoumpas C, Buerger C, King AP, et al. Fast generation of 4D PET-MR data from real dynamic MR acquisitions. Phys Med Biol 2011;56(20):6597–613.

58. Baumgartner CF, Kolbitsch C, Balfour DR, et al. High-resolution dynamic MR imaging of the thorax for respiratory motion correction of PET using group wise manifold alignment. Med Image Anal 2014;18(7):939–52.

59. Fayad HJ, Odille F, Felblinger J, et al. A generic PET/MRI respiratory motion correction using a generalized reconstruction by inversion of coupled systems (GRICS) approach. IEEE Nuclear Science Symposium and Medical Imaging Conference (NSS/MIC). October 27 – November 3, 2012. p. 2813–6.

60. Buerger C, Schaeffter T, King AP. Hierarchical adaptive local affine registration for fast and robust

respiratory motion estimation. Med Image Anal 2011;15:551–64.

61. King AP, Buerger C, Tsoumpas C, et al. Thoracic respiratory motion estimation from MRI using a statistical model and a 2-D image navigator. Med Image Anal 2012;16(1):252–64.

62. Buerger C, Tsoumpas C, Aitken A, et al. Investigation of MR-based attenuation correction and motion compensation for hybrid PET/MR. IEEE Trans Nucl Sci 2012;59(5):1967–76.

63. Liang D, Liu B, Wang J, et al. Accelerating SENSE using compressed sensing. Magn Reson Med 2009;62(6):1574–84.

64. Fayad H, Odille F, Schmidt H, et al. The use of a generalized reconstruction by inversion of coupled systems (GRICS) approach for generic respiratory motion correction in PET/MR imaging. Phys Med Biol 2015;60(6):2529–46.

65. Weissler B, Gebhardt P, Lerche CW, et al. PET/MR synchronization by detection of switching gradients. IEEE Trans Nucl Sci 2015;62(3):650–7.

66. Fieseler M, Kugel H, Gigengack F, et al. A dynamic thorax phantom for the assessment of cardiac and respiratory motion correction in PET/MRI: a preliminary evaluation. Nucl Instrum Methods Phys Res A 2013;702:59–63.

67. Soultanidis GM, Mackewn JE, Tsoumpas C, et al. PVA cryogel for construction of deformable PET-MR visible phantoms. IEEE Trans Nucl Sci 2013; 60(1):95–102.

68. Polycarpou I, Tsoumpas C, Marsden PK. Analysis and comparison of two methods for motion correction in PET imaging. Med Phys 2012;39:6474–83.

69. Tsoumpas C, Polycarpou I, Thielemans K, et al. The effect of regularization in motion compensated PET image reconstruction: a realistic numerical 4D simulation study. Phys Med Biol 2013;58:1759–73.

70. Chun SY, Fessler JA. Spatial resolution properties of motion-compensated tomographic image reconstruction methods. IEEE Trans Med Imaging 2012; 31:1413–25.

71. Thielemans K, Tsoumpas C, Mustafovic S, et al. STIR: software for tomographic image reconstruction release 2. Phys Med Biol 2012;57(4):867–83.

72. Fayad H, Schmidt H, Würslin C, et al. Reconstruction incorporated respiratory motion correction in clinical simultaneous PET/MR imaging for oncology applications. J Nucl Med 2015;56(6):884–9.

73. Manber R, Thielemans K, Hutton B, et al. Practical PET respiratory motion correction in clinical PET/MR. J Nucl Med 2015;56(6):890–6.

74. Catana C. Motion correction options in PET/MRI. Semin Nucl Med 2015;45(3):212–23.

75. Izquierdo D, Catana C. Magnetic resonance imaging-guided attenuation correction of positron emission tomography data in PET/MRI. PET Clin, in press.

76. Samarin A, Burger C, Wollenweber SD, et al. PET/MR imaging of bone lesions—implications for PET quantification from imperfect attenuation correction. Eur J Nucl Med Mol Imaging 2012;39:1154–60.

77. Eiber M, Martinez-Möller A, Souvatzoglou M, et al. Value of a Dixon-based MR/PET attenuation correction sequence for the localization and evaluation of PET-positive lesions. Eur J Nucl Med Mol Imaging 2011;38:1691–701.

78. Kong E, Cho I. Clinical issues regarding misclassification by Dixon based PET/MR attenuation correction. Hell J Nucl Med 2015;18(1):42–7.

79. Schleyer PJ, Schaeffter T, Marsden PK. The effect of inaccurate bone attenuation coefficient and segmentation on reconstructed PET images. Nucl Med Commun 2010;31(8):708–16.

80. Keereman V, Fierens Y, Broux T, et al. MRI-based attenuation correction for PET/MRI using ultrashort echo time sequences. J Nucl Med 2010;51:812–8.

81. Chang EY, Du J, Chung CB. UTE imaging in the musculoskeletal system. J Magn Reson Imaging 2015;41:870–83.

82. Monnier F, Fayad H, Bert J, et al. Clinical MR-based attenuation correction using continuous linear attenuation coefficients derived from a simple Dixon-like sequence. J Nucl Med 2015;56:1795.

83. Hofmann M, Steinke F, Scheel V, et al. MRI-based attenuation correction for PET/MRI: a novel approach combining pattern recognition and atlas registration. J Nucl Med 2008;49(11):1875–83.

84. Burgos N, Cardoso MJ, Thielemans K, et al. Attenuation correction synthesis for hybrid PET-MR scanners: application to brain studies. IEEE Trans Med Imaging 2014;33(12):2332–41.

85. Ladefoged CN, Benoit D, Law I, et al. PET/MR attenuation correction in brain imaging using a continuous bone signal derived from UTE. 4th Conf on PET/MR and SPECT/MR. Elba Isle, Italy, May 17–20, 2015.

86. Defrise M, Rezaei A, Nuyts J. Time-of-flight PET data determine the attenuation sinogram up to a constant. Phys Med Biol 2012;57(4):885.

87. Mehranian A, Zaidi H. Impact of time-of-flight PET on quantification errors in MRI-based attenuation correction. J Nucl Med 2015;56(4):635–41.

88. Watson CC. Supplemental transmission method for improved PET attenuation correction on an integrated MR/PET. Nucl Instrum Methods Phys Res A 2014;734:191–5.

89. Mollet P, Keereman V, Bini J, et al. Improvement of attenuation correction in time-of-flight PET/MR imaging with a positron-emitting source. J Nucl Med 2014;55(2):329–36.

90. Rothfuss H, Panin V, Hong I, et al. LSO background radiation as a transmission source using time of flight information. Phys Med Biol 2014;59(18): 5483–500.

91. Watson CC. Extension of single scatter simulation to scatter correction of time-of-flight PET. IEEE Trans Nucl Sci 2007;54(5):1679–86.

92. Thielemans K, Manjeshwar RM, Tsoumpas C, et al. A new algorithm for scaling of PET scatter estimates using all coincidence events. IEEE Nuclear Science Symposium Conference Record, NSS 2007 (Volume: 5). October 26 – November 3, 2007. p. 3586–90.

93. Zaidi H, Montandon M-L, Alavi A. Advances in attenuation correction techniques in PET. PET Clin 2007;2(2):191–217.

94. Prasad R, Zaidi H. A cone-shaped phantom for assessment of small animal PET scatter fraction and count rate performance. Mol Imaging Biol 2012;14(5):561–71.

95. Cheng JC, Boellaard R, Laforest R. Evaluation of the effect of magnetic field on PET spatial resolution and contrast recovery using clinical PET scanners and EGSnrc simulations. IEEE Trans Nucl Sci 2015;62(1):101–10.

96. Iida H, Kanno I, Miura S, et al. A simulation study of a method to reduce positron annihilation spread distributions using a strong magnetic field in positron emission tomography. IEEE Trans Nucl Sci 1986;33(1):597–600.

97. Shah NJ, Herzog H, Weirich C, et al. Effects of magnetic fields of up to 9.4 T on resolution and contrast of PET images as measured with an MR-BrainPET. PLoS One 2014;9(4):e95250.

98. Kraus R, Delso G, Ziegler S. Simulation study of tissue-specific positron range correction for the new biograph mMR whole-body PET/MR system. IEEE Trans Nucl Sci 2012;59(5):1900–9.

99. Bertolli O, Cecchetti M, Camarlinghi N, et al. Iterative reconstruction incorporating positron range correction within STIR framework. Eur J Nucl Med Mol Imag Phys 2014;1(1):A42.

100. Fung EK, Carson RE. Cerebral blood flow with [15O] water PET studies using an image-derived input function and MR-defined carotid centerlines. Phys Med Biol 2013;58:1903–23.

101. Bousse A, Pedemonte S, Thomas BA, et al. Markov random field and Gaussian mixture for segmented MRI-based partial volume correction in PET. Phys Med Biol 2012;57(20):6681–705.

102. Petibon Y, Huang C, Ouyang J, et al. Relative role of motion and PSF compensation in whole-body oncologic PET-MR imaging. Med Phys 2014; 41(4):042503.

103. Fessler JA, Clinthorne NH, Rogers WL. Regularized emission image reconstruction using imperfect side information. IEEE Trans Nucl Sci 1992;39(5):1464–71.

104. Gindi GL, Lee M, Rangarajan A, et al. Bayesian reconstruction of functional images using anatomical information as priors. IEEE Trans Med Imaging 1993;2(4):670–80.

105. Ouyang X, Wong WH, Johnson VE, et al. Incorporation of correlated structural images in PET image reconstruction. IEEE Trans Med Imaging 1994; 13(4):627–40.

106. Vunckx K, Nuyts J. Heuristic modification of an anatomical Markov prior improves its performance. IEEE Nuclear Science Symposium Conference Record (NSS/MIC). October 30 – November 6, 2010. p. 3262–66.

107. Bowsher JE, Hong Y, Hedlund LW, et al. Utilizing MRI information to estimate F18-FDG distributions in rat flank tumors. IEEE Nuclear Science Symposium Conference Record, (Volume: 4), October 16–22, 2004. p. 2488–92.

108. Karaoglanis K, Gaitanis A, Tsoumpas C. Evaluation of modified median root prior on a myocardium study, using realistic PET/MR data. IEEE 13th International Conference on Bioinformatics and Bioengineering (BIBE), November 10–13, 2013.

109. Caldeira CL, Scheins J, Almeida P, et al. Evaluation of two methods for using MR information in PET reconstruction. Nucl Instrum Methods Phys Res A 2013;702:141–3.

110. Loeb R, Navab N, Ziegler S. Direct parametric reconstruction using anatomical regularization for simultaneous PET/MRI data. IEEE Trans Med Imaging 2015;34(11):2233–47.

111. Iguchi S, Hori Y, Moriguchi T, et al. Verification of a semi-automated MRI-guided technique for noninvasive determination of the arterial input function in 15O-labeled gaseous PET. Nucl Instrum Methods Phys Res A 2013;702:111–3.

112. Chun SY, Reese TG, Ouyang J, et al. MRI-based nonrigid motion correction in simultaneous PET/MRI. J Nucl Med 2012;53:1284–91.

113. de Rosales RTM, Tavare R, Paul RL, et al. Synthesis of Cu-64(II)-Bis(dithiocarbamatebisphosphonate) and its conjugation with superparamagnetic iron oxide nanoparticles: in vivo evaluation as dual-modality PET-MRI agent. Angew Chem Int Ed Engl 2011;50(24):5509–13.

The Use of Contrast Agents in Clinical and Preclinical PET-MR Imaging

Lydia Sandiford, PhD, Rafael T.M. de Rosales, PhD*

KEYWORDS

• PET-MR imaging • Contrast agents • Imaging agents • Bimodal imaging agents

KEY POINTS

- Contrast agents (CAs) can be used in two ways in clinical and preclinical PET-MR imaging: (i) an unimodal approach and (ii) in a bimodal approach.
- The bimodal approach adds better quantification and whole-body detectability to MR imaging CAs.
- Radiolabeling of responsive MR imaging contrast agents and the use of PET-MRI allows for quantification, which is a requirement for accurate measurements.

INTRODUCTION

PET-MR imaging has the major advantage of combining two medical imaging modalities that can provide highly complementary multiparametric information with low radiation doses (compared with PET-computed tomography [CT]) and the possibility of simultaneous acquisitions. To exploit this synergy fully, researchers in the clinical and preclinical fields have the possibility of exploiting the several contrast agents (CAs) available, clinically and preclinically, for each technique as well as the possibility of combining them into a single, bimodal CA. Each approach has its advantages and disadvantages and we discuss them herein. However, to fully appreciate them we should first look at an overview of the inherent properties of PET and MR imaging CAs separately.

Contrast Agents in MR imaging

To obtain contrast, the use of paramagnetic metals such as gadolinium and iron, which alter the relaxation properties of water, is required. At the moment there are only 5 CAs that have been approved by the US Food and Drug Administration based on gadolinium: gadopentetate dimeglumine (Magnevist), gadobenate dimeglumine (MultiHance), gadodiamide (Omniscan), gadoversetamide (OptiMARK), and gadoteridol (ProHance). All of these CAs are not targeted and are mainly used to increase the contrast of blood and hence are only useful used to image vasculature and its abnormalities, mainly in the central nervous system. A major advantage of contrast-enhanced MR imaging techniques is their high spatial and temporal resolution, allowing the visualization of very small capillaries and areas of high perfusion.

The second class of MR imaging CAs is based on colloidal suspensions of superparamagnetic inorganic materials based on iron oxides, commonly termed as superparamagnetic iron oxide (SPIO) nanoparticles. These materials are composed of single nanoparticles and/or aggregates, coated with an organic coating, such as

The authors acknowledge financial support from The Centre of Excellence in Medical Engineering funded by the Wellcome Trust and EPSRC under Grant No. WT 088641/Z/09/Z. and the Department of Health via the National Institute for Health Research (NIHR) comprehensive Biomedical Research Center award to Guy's & St Thomas' NHS Foundation Trust in partnership with King's College London and King's College Hospital NHS Foundation Trust.
Division of Imaging Sciences and Biomedical Engineering, King's College London, St. Thomas' Hospital, London SE1 7EH, UK
* Corresponding author.
E-mail address: rafael.torres@kcl.ac.uk

PET Clin 11 (2016) 119–128
http://dx.doi.org/10.1016/j.cpet.2015.10.003
1556-8598/16/$ – see front matter © 2016 Elsevier Inc. All rights reserved.

carbohydrates or polyethylene glycol polymers, that prevent aggregation of the inorganic material as well as serving as potential targeting agents (eg, macrophage uptake enhanced by carbohydrate coatings). The main use of SPIOs in the clinic has been in the detection using imaging of lesions of the liver such as tumors, because they do not readily take up SPIO CAs, resulting in significant contrast with the surrounding tissue. In the preclinical field, SPIOs have also been extensively used for cell labeling and tracking using MR imaging as well as for tumor imaging by exploiting the enhanced permeation and retention effect of some tumors or by the attachment of tumor-targeting targeting vectors (eg, antibodies, peptides).[1,2] Many preclinical studies have also exploited the hyperthermic properties of these materials for tumor treatment.[1,3]

The major disadvantage of MR imaging CAs is related to the inherently low sensitivity of MR imaging, meaning that, to obtain contrast, large amounts of paramagnetic ions are required. For example, for a 70-kg subject the typical dose of gadolinium is between 1 and 2 g. This amount represents a significant toxicity risk for patients, because this amount of free gadolinium ions may be toxic and indeed it has been shown that patients with impaired excretion function are prone to suffer from its deleterious effects leading to nephrogenic systemic fibrosis. In addition, although rare, the use of gadolinium CAs have resulted in life-threatening anaphylactic and anaphylactoid reactions. In the search of safer and more efficient MR imaging CAs, there is a substantial effort to generate MR imaging CAs with higher relaxivity (a measure of how efficient CAs relax water molecules and hence of signal/CA molecule) by means of increasing the number of gadolinium/Fe per CA molecule or by modulating their relaxation properties.[4] To date, however, none of these have resulted in a change or increase in the clinical use of MR imaging CAs. A second challenge is related to quantification, a key concept in molecular imaging, and most likely the reason of the limited interest for molecular imaging using MR imaging CAs. The reasons behind this are beyond the scope of this review but, compared with nuclear imaging techniques such as PET (vide infra), where absolute in vivo quantification is possible and relatively simple to achieve, it is very challenging and time consuming to quantify the amount of CAs using MR imaging.

Contrast Agents in PET

In this imaging modality, CAs rely on the use of positron emitting radionuclides produced in either biomedical cyclotrons (eg, ^{18}F, ^{11}C, ^{13}N, ^{64}Cu, [89]Zr) or generators (eg, [82]Rb, ^{68}Ga). PET radiotracers may be composed of just the radionuclide itself (eg, [82]Rb) or more commonly attached to a molecule via a covalent bond or covalent coordinate bonds in the case of radiometals. Once inside the body, PET radiotracers are detected by the scanner providing information of their location and concentration in different tissues. One of the main differences with MR imaging CAs is the larger amount of PET tracers available for clinical use. This is most likely the result of their lower toxicity risk, a consequence of the higher sensitivity, defined as the amount of imaging agent required to obtain contrast, of PET imaging compared with MR imaging. The only toxicity risk for these agents is owing to their radioactive properties, but these are usually very low and measurable. The most used agent in PET is fluorodeoxyglucose (^{18}F-FDG), a tracer useful to image glucose-avid tissues that has found wide applications in tumor and inflammation imaging.[5] However, unlike for MR imaging where clinical CAs have limited applications, PET tracers are available that image completely different biological projects. For example, ^{18}F-fluoride has high affinity to hydroxyapatite, which is the main component of bone and calcified tissues, making it useful to image bone metabolism and vascular calcifications.[6] Information about disease-related cell receptors and their concentrations in tissues is also available in PET by using radiolabeled peptides such as arginine-glycine-aspartic (RGD; angiogenesis) and octreotride (neuroendocrine tumors) using ^{18}F or ^{68}Ga, or antibodies such as trastuzumab (HER2 receptor) using [89]Zr or [64]Cu.[7,8]

CONTRAST AGENTS IN PET-MR IMAGING STUDIES (CLINICAL AND PRECLINICAL)

In PET-MR imaging we have the advantage that we can use CAs in both techniques as well as the option of using bimodal CAs. Thus, we could classify the use of CAs in PET-MR imaging in two methods:

- *Unimodal approach*. CAs for one of both techniques, given nonsimultaneously or simultaneously (cocktail), are used to obtain multiparametric information.
- *Bimodal approach*. A bimodal imaging agent is generated with the goal of providing an enhanced CA for a specific purpose.

There are specific applications for each approach and each one has advantages and disadvantages.[9] The first one is quickly translatable from the preclinical to the clinical arena, providing we are using clinically approved CAs, and also has the advantage of providing different types of information, from a single imaging session. The second approach, currently at the preclinical evaluation stage, is aimed at enhancing the properties of a given CA with a second modality component. For reasons we described in a recent minireview,[10] it is only feasible to develop bimodal PET-MR imaging agents based in the radiolabeling of an MR CA and, by doing so, adding the excellent quantification and whole-body detectability properties of PET (vide infra).

Unimodal Approach

There are many examples of the use of multiple CAs in PET-MR imaging studies and how they can be used to obtain multiparametric information for a more accurate diagnosis or to monitor treatment response. A common theme in these studies is the use of contrast-enhanced MR imaging as well as other sequences to identify areas of high and low perfusion or vascularity and PET tracers to provide functional information (eg, angiogenesis, glucose metabolism). In the cardiology field,

an elegant example is given by Makowski and colleagues,[11] in which a patient that had suffered from myocardial infarction and had been treated by percutaneous coronary intervention (angioplasty with a stent) underwent an MR imaging and PET-CT imaging study (**Fig. 1**). MR imaging using gadopentetic acid (Gd-DTPA) indicated scar tissue by delayed enhancement in areas of the left ventricle. In addition, ^{13}N-NH$_3$ (^{13}N-ammonia), a PET tracer that is taken up by cells of viable tissue by means of the ammonia transporter, identified areas of low perfusion that corresponded to the scar tissue in the Gd-DTPA MR imaging. Interestingly, the authors also evaluated the use of a radiolabeled peptide, ^{18}F-galacto-RGD, that binds to the $\alpha_v\beta_3$ integrin, a cell receptor overexpressed in angiogenic tissues. The study revealed uptake in the same areas where the Gd-DTPA MR imaging and ^{13}N-NH$_3$ studies showed scar tissue and low perfusion, suggesting angiogenesis. The authors conclude this may be an indication of an underlying healing process in the affected area. It would be interesting to see how this type of multiparametric imaging study correlates with long-term outcomes.

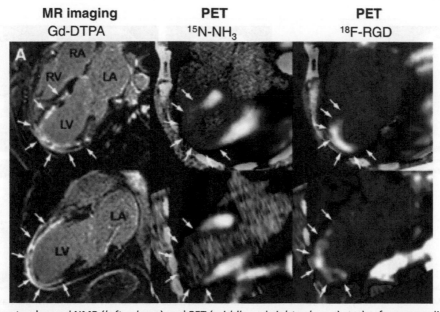

MR imaging   **PET**   **PET**
Gd-DTPA ^{15}N-NH$_3$ ^{18}F-RGD

Fig. 1. Contrast-enhanced NMR (*left column*) and PET (*middle and right columns*) study of a myocardial infraction patient with delayed enhancement (*arrows*) extending from the anterior wall to the apical region in the 4-chamber (*top row*) and 2-chamber (*bottom row*) views. (*Middle column*) Identically reproduced location and geometry with severely reduced myocardial blood flow using ^{13}N-ammonia, corresponding to the regions of delayed enhancement by contrast-enhanced (Gd-DTPA) NMR (*left column, arrows*). (*Right column*) Focal ^{18}F-RGD signal colocalized to the infarcted area, reflecting the extent of the $\alpha_v\beta_3$ expression. This signal may reflect angiogenesis within the healing area (*arrows*). LA, left atrium; LV, left ventricle; RA, right atrium; RV, right ventricle. (*Adapted from* Makowski MR, Ebersberger U, Nekolla S, et al. In vivo molecular imaging of angiogenesis, targeting alphavbeta3 integrin expression, in a patient after acute myocardial infarction. Eur Heart J 2008;29(18):2201; with permission.)

Another interesting application is in the study of brain tumors owing to the lack of anatomic detail and sensitivity of CT in this area. For example, a comparison between ^{18}F-FDG PET-CT and ^{18}F-FDG PET-MR imaging showed how the combination of MR imaging and PET allowed the detection of small cerebral metastases that PET-CT or PET did not detect (**Fig. 2**). Thus, the contrast-enhanced MR imaging allows the detection of sub-centimeter cerebral metastases, confirmed by areas of high ^{18}F-FDG PET, whereas the same lesions where not detected by PET, CT, or PET-CT alone.[12] Similarly, another study showed how the combination of contrast-enhanced MR imaging and ^{18}F-FDG PET allowed for the identification of a sarcoma metastases in a muscle that was not clearly identified by contrast-enhanced CT (**Fig. 3**).[13] These 2 examples highlight the synergy between PET, MR imaging, and the use of CAs that may allow for more accurate staging and diagnoses and for the efficient preoperative planning of operative procedures.

The use of ^{68}Ga in PET, particularly for labeling peptides, is experiencing an increasing interest owing to its availability from a clinical grade generator and examples in the field of oncologic PET-MR imaging are starting to emerge. For example,

Afshar-Oromich and colleagues[14] used a ^{68}Ga-PSMA (prostate-specific membrane antigen) radiotracer to locate metastatic sentinel lymph nodes (SLNs) and the areas in the prostate of a cancer patient of high uptake and used T2-weighted MR imaging and apparent diffusion coefficient maps to provide further anatomic and functional information for a more diagnostic accuracy. This is a good example showing how MR imaging can not only provide excellent anatomic soft tissue information, but also exploit its versatility to deliver functional information without the need of CAs (eg, diffusion-weighted imaging).

In the preclinical field, the use of combined CAs for PET-MR imaging has been mainly restricted to oncologic studies. A pioneering study by Judenhofer and colleagues[15] demonstrated how the use of the 2 imaging modalities as well as CAs allowed to explain the radiotracer's tumor uptake heterogeneity commonly found in PET studies. In this report, the authors studied a CT26 colon carcinoma mouse model using ^{18}F-FLT (3'-deoxy-3'-^{18}F-fluorothymidine), a radiotracer that may be useful to image tumor proliferation using a preclinical PET-MR imaging scanner. The PET image clearly showed areas of high uptake that correspond with areas of high

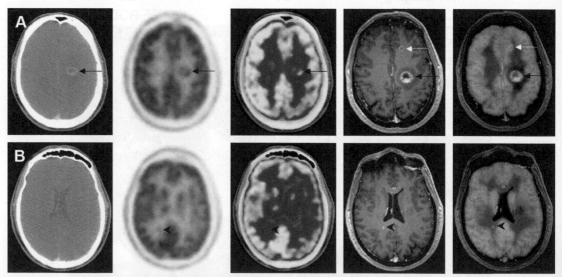

Fig. 2. PET-MR imaging study of a patient with cerebral metastases from cancer of unknown primary. (A) Large left hemisphere metastasis (*black arrow*) is visible on (from *left to right*) axial contrast-enhanced computed tomography (CT), ^{18}F-FDG PET, PET-CT, axial contrast-enhanced MR imaging, and PET-MR imaging, whereas smaller metastasis of left frontal lobe (*white arrow*) is visible solely on MR imaging and PET-MR imaging. Location of this metastasis directly adjacent to highly ^{18}F-FDG–avid cortex leads to problems with diagnosing this lesion on ^{18}F-FDG PET scan. (B) Another subcentimeter-sized metastasis of right temporal lobe, clearly visible on MR imaging and PET-MR imaging of same patient (*arrowhead*), was only retrospectively seen as faintly increased ^{18}F-FDG activity on PET and PET-CT because of lack of anatomic correlate on CT. (This research was originally published in *JNM*. Buchbender C, Heusner TA, Lauenstein TC, et al. Oncologic PET/MR imaging, part 1: tumors of the brain, head and neck, chest, abdomen, and pelvis. J Nucl Med 2012;53(6):928–38. © by the Society of Nuclear Medicine and Molecular Imaging, Inc.)

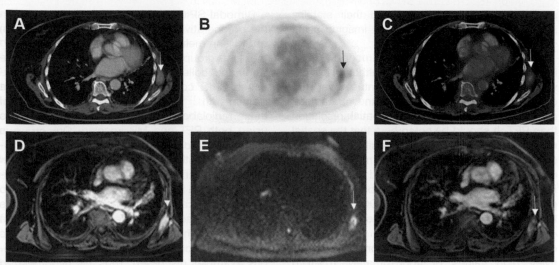

Fig. 3. PET-MR imaging study of a patient with sarcoma metastasis in left anterior serratus muscle. Axial contrast-enhanced computed tomography (CT) scan (*A*) shows ill-defined muscle-isodense soft tissue mass (*arrow*) that is ^{18}F-FDG–avid on ^{18}F-FDG PET (*B*) and ^{18}F-FDG PET-CT (*C*). Extent of this mass is better depicted on axial contrast-enhanced fat-suppressed MR imaging (*D*). Diffusion-weighted MR image (*E*) depicts this metastasis as high-signal diffusion-restricted lesion (*arrow*) and demonstrates sensitivity of diffusion-weighted MR imaging. ^{18}F -FDG PET-MR image is also shown (*F*). (This research was originally published in *JNM*. Buchbender C, Heusner TA, Lauenstein TC, et al. Oncologic PET/MRI, part 2: bone tumors, soft-tissue tumors, melanoma, and lymphoma. J Nucl Med 2012;53(8):1244–52. © by the Society of Nuclear Medicine and Molecular Imaging, Inc.)

cell proliferation. The question that remains is whether the areas of low uptake are necrotic or do they correspond with nonproliferating cancer cells? By looking at the dynamic MR imaging and the pre– and post–contrast-enhanced MR imaging profiles of the tumor, the authors were able to correlate areas of low ^{18}F-FLT uptake with areas of low perfusion and areas of necrosis and inflammation.

As mentioned, PET-MR imaging allows for the collection of multiparametric information, potentially from a single imaging session. This advantage has been exploited by Viel and colleagues[16] while studying the dynamics of growth of glioblastomas in animal models. The authors followed the tumors for up 6 weeks using a combination of PET (^{18}F-FDG, ^{18}F-FLT, and ^{11}C-MET) and MR imaging (T2-weighted and contrast-enhanced T1-weighted images). ^{11}C-MET (L-[methyl-^{11}C]methionine) is another short-lived PET tracer ($t_{1/2}$ - ^{11}C = 20.3 min) useful to image tumors that show an increase in methionine uptake. It was found that both ^{18}F-FLT and ^{11}C-MET detected tumors earlier than ^{18}F-FDG, partly owing to the high intrinsic uptake of this tracer in brain tissue. Interestingly, the uptake of ^{11}C-MET was an early indicator of proliferation and vessel permeability. In addition, MR imaging using a combination of both T2-weighted and contrast-enhanced T1-weighted sequences allowed the identification and accurate delineation of the tumors at late stages of tumor development, which could be useful for surgery and/or radiotherapy planning of these types of tumors.

Bimodal Approach

All the current examples reported to date in this category are in the synthesis and developmental stage without a focused potential clinical application and some are in the preclinical stage. As we alluded to, the most logical use of this approach is to add a radionuclide component to an MR CA, hence providing:

1. Better quantification (PET vs MR imaging), and
2. Better whole body detectability, for guiding high-resolution MR imaging.

The majority of reports of bimodal PET-MR imaging CAs started appearing in the scientific literature in 2008. Nahrendorf and colleagues[17] modified a dextran-coated SPIO with a DTPA chelator for successfully imaging macrophage-rich atherosclerotic plaque in a mouse model (Apolipoprotein E$^{-/-}$) using ^{64}Cu for PET. Another similar method to generate ^{64}Cu-labeled dextran-coated SPIOs was reported in the same year by Jarret and colleagues[18] using DOTA, a chelator that is known to form more kinetically inert complexes with copper than DTPA. Using a different strategy, Glaus and colleagues[19] radiolabeled micelle-coated SPIOs using DOTA-conjugated phospholipids and demonstrated their stability and potential for in vivo PET-MR imaging using standard BALB/c mice.

Several groups have explored bimodal PET-MR imaging agents to image tumors, although it is not yet clear what would be the advantage over PET CAs beyond being able to locate the intratumoral areas of uptake with higher spatial resolution than PET. It should be noted here that the spatial resolution of clinical PET is quite high when compared with previous nuclear medicine techniques. Lee and colleagues[20] used an SPIO scaffold to functionalize the nanoparticles using polyaspartic acid anchors with DOTA chelators for ^{64}Cu binding as well as RGD peptides integrin $\alpha_v\beta_3$ targeting. In vitro and in vivo studies confirmed specific binding to tumor reaching relatively high values of approximately 10%ID/g (**Fig. 4**). The specificity of the probe toward $\alpha_v\beta_3$ receptors was confirmed in blocking studies. Xie and colleagues[21] used a different strategy. This group used dopamine to coat the surface of SPIOs with albumin using standard bioconjugation techniques, followed by conjugation with ^{64}Cu-DOTA and a fluorophore. The resulting trimodal CA was successfully used to image the U87MG xenograft mouse model by exploiting the enhanced permeation and retention effect.[21]

Bimodal SPIOs have great clinical potential in the preoperative localization and characterization of SLNs in melanoma and breast cancer. Among the first groups to explore this concept were Choi and colleagues,[22] who used an albumin-based SPIO coating approach to radiolabel the protein with [124]I, and demonstrated the utility of these radiolabeled SPIOs to image SLNs in vivo using both PET and MR imaging. Our group is very interested in this application and we approached it with a different strategy to radiolabel SPIOs. We started with the premise of using clinically approved SPIOs such as Endorem/Feridex to facilitate clinical translation. However, we were interested in radiolabeling techniques that did not require any chemical reaction with the organic coating component of the SPIOs, as in the previous examples discussed. Thus, we hypothesized that using a small bifunctional metallic complex with high affinity for both the radionuclide and the inorganic surface of the nanoparticle may allow us to radiolabel SPIOs in a way that did not affect its physicochemical properties. Thus, using small bifunctional bisphosphonates we were able to radiolabel Endorem/Feridex, as well as other inorganic-based nanoparticles for imaging, with ^{64}Cu and other radionuclides in high yields and with high in vitro and in vivo stability.[23–26]

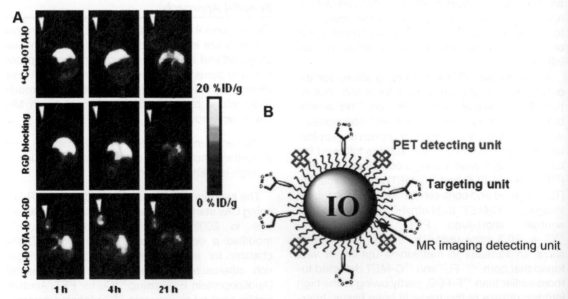

Fig. 4. (*A*) Decay-corrected whole-body coronal PET images of nude mouse bearing human U87MG tumor at 1, 4, and 21 hours after injection of 3.7 MBq of ^{64}Cu-DOTA-iron oxide nanoparticles (IO), ^{64}Cu-DOTA-IO-RGD, or ^{64}Cu-DOTA-IO-RGD with 10 mg of c(RGDyK) peptide per kilogram (300 μg of iron-equivalent IO particles per mouse). (*B*) Structure of ^{64}Cu-DOTA-IO-RGD nanoparticles. (This research was originally published in *JNM*. Lee HY, Li Z, Chen K, et al. PET/MRI dual-modality tumor imaging using arginine-glycine-aspartic (RGD)-conjugated radiolabeled iron oxide nanoparticles. J Nucl Med 2008;49(8):1371–9. © by the Society of Nuclear Medicine and Molecular Imaging, Inc.)

Furthermore, preclinical PET/MR imaging studies confirmed their potential for SLN imaging studies in a nontumor model (**Fig. 5**).[24] In more recent studies, Madru and colleagues[27] and Thorek and colleagues[28] have also explored the same SLN bimodal imaging concept using ^{99m}Tc and ^{89}Zr, respectively, by radiolabeling the organic coating of SPIOs.

Another interesting approach to generate multimodal nanoparticles is by incorporating the PET radiometal during SPIO synthesis, usually using the thermal decomposition method, or by direct activation using a cyclotron (**Fig. 6**). These radiolabeling methods are potentially useful for studying the fate and metabolism of inorganic nanoparticles in preclinical studies, but have limited applications in a clinical setting, where radiochemical speed and reproducibility are essential requirements. Chakravarty and colleagues[29] have successfully incorporated the PET radionuclide ^{69}Ge ($t\sqrt{2}$ = 39.05 h, 21% β^+, E_{max} = 1205 keV) into SPIOs and demonstrated their stability and potential use for SLN imaging using PET-MR imaging. Similar methods can be used to incorporate ^{59}Fe and ^{52}Mn into SPIOs as recently shown by Freund and colleagues[30] and Hoffman and colleagues,[31] respectively.

There are fewer reports of bimodal agents based in small gadolinium compounds for combined T1-weighted MR imaging–PET imaging. In the nanoparticle field an interesting approach

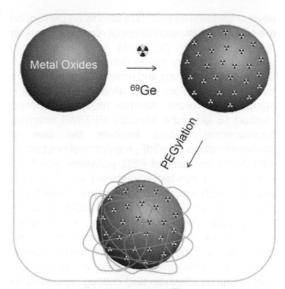

Fig. 6. Chelator-free synthesis of ^{69}Ge-metal oxides for multimodal imaging. (*Adapted from* Chakravarty R, Valdovinos HF, Chen F, et al. Intrinsically germanium-69-labeled iron oxide nanoparticles: synthesis and in-vivo dual-modality PET/MR imaging. Adv Mater 2014;26(30):5120; with permission.)

reported by Truillet and colleagues[32] exploits a novel nanoparticle platform based on a polysiloxane matrix that yields nanoparticles of extremely small and monodispersed size, capable of being cleared by the renal pathway while allowing

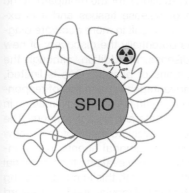

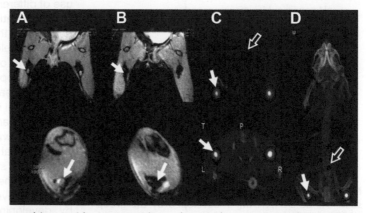

Fig. 5. (*Left*) Radiolabeling of dextran-coated iron oxide nanoparticles such as Endorem using radiolabeled bisphosphonates (BPs). (*Right*) In vivo PET–MR imaging studies with [^{64}Cu(dtcbp)$_2$]–Endorem in a mouse. (*A, B*) Coronal (*top*) and short axis (*bottom*) MR images of the lower abdominal area and upper hind legs showing the popliteal lymph nodes (*solid arrows*) before (*A*) and after (*B*) footpad injection of [^{64}Cu(dtcbp)$_2$]–Endorem. (*C*) Coronal (*top*) and short-axis (*bottom*) NanoPET–CT images of the same mouse as in (*B*) showing the uptake of [^{64}Cu(dtcbp)$_2$]–Endorem in the popliteal (*solid arrow*) and iliac lymph nodes (*hollow arrow*). (*D*) Whole-body NanoPET–CT images showing sole uptake of [^{64}Cu(dtcbp)$_2$]–Endorem in the popliteal and iliac lymph nodes. No translocation of radioactivity to other tissues was detected. SPIO, superparamagnetic iron oxide. (*Adapted from* de Rosales RTM, Tavare R, Paul RL, et al. Synthesis of Cu-64(II)-Bis(dithiocarbamatebisphosphonate) and its conjugation with superparamagnetic iron oxide nanoparticles: in vivo evaluation as dual-modality PET-MRI agent. Angew Chem Int Ed Engl 2011;50(24):5508; with permission.)

several gadolinium and ^{68}Ga ions to be present on the surface. This yields bimodal nanoparticles with high r_1 relaxivity (10.3 mM^{-1}s^{-1}) and in vivo studies in a healthy mouse demonstrated colocalization of both signals and renal excretion. It will be interesting to explore this platform for targeted imaging in the future. Another recently proposed method to generate trimodal (PET/MR imaging/fluorescence) agents involves the use of lanthanide-doped NaGdF$_4$ nanophosphors coated with a combination of PEG polymers and RGD peptides that can be radiolabeled with [124]I using standard radioiodination techniques.[33] Preclinical studies in an integrin-positive U87MG tumor model using this CA have shown promising results, but questions remain open about the potential toxicity of these lanthanide-rich nanomaterials.

In the small molecule field, most of the work has been done by Caravan and colleagues and Aime and colleagues using pH-responsive MR imaging CAs based in small gadolinium complexes and metallic radionuclides. MR imaging CAs can be designed to be responsive (ie, CA changes relaxivity or 'signal intensity') to external factors such as pH, which is a potential biomarker of tumors.[34] However, to provide accurate measurements, it is a requirement to know the concentration of the CA in the tissue of interest. To do this with MR imaging, particularly in areas of low or high uptake, is a very challenging task. A solution to this problem is to add a radionuclide reporter that allows quantification and increases its detectability. Thus, these imaging agents (**Fig. 7**) comprise 2 reporters: a gadolinium-based MR imaging reporter that changes its relaxivity (the "signal intensity") with pH, and a radionuclide that provides the sensitivity and quantification properties. This radionuclide can be added to the organic molecule by standard fluorination (^{18}F) chemistry,[35] or by exchanging some of the gadolinium atoms with a radiometal such as [166]Ho.[36]

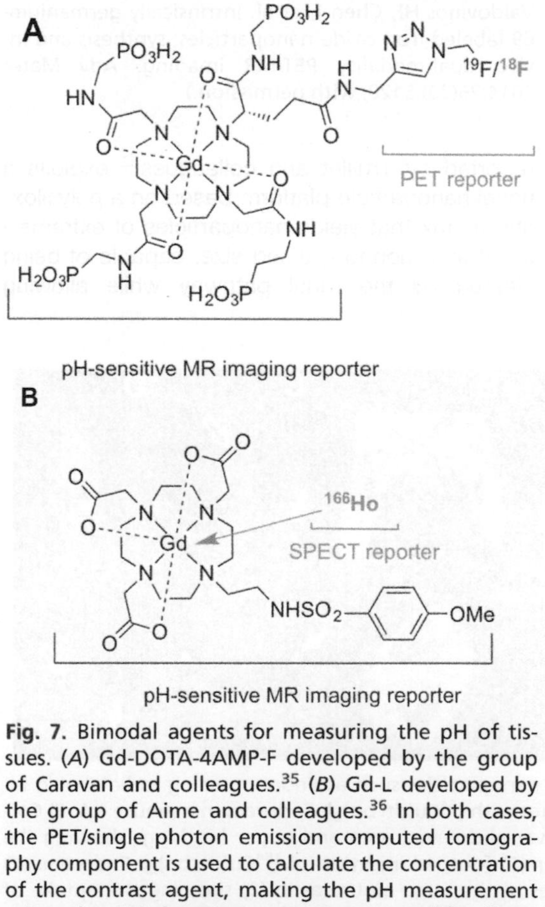

SUMMARY

PET-MR imaging is now entering the clinical field and many scanners have been already installed worldwide. It is expected that this number will increase gradually and many hospitals will adopt this hybrid technique with clear advantages in several important areas (eg, pediatric, central nervous system, cardiovascular, and oncology). The use of different CAs allows for the multiparametric characterization of disease tissues and it is expected that this may result in more accurate diagnoses as well as potentially the discovery of new biomarkers of disease. In addition, although the potential applications of bimodal CAs is limited, there are clear advantages in the fields of responsive bimodal MR imaging CAs and SLN imaging in melanoma, and prostate and breast cancers. The next stage will be to evaluate some of these new CA combinations and bimodal agents in first-in-man clinical studies to fully evaluate their potential to improve health care. With this in mind, imaging chemists have the task of moving the field forward by developing novel synthetic techniques and translate them into clinically useful radiotracers and MR imaging CAs that will likely result in many new applications in the future.

Fig. 7. Bimodal agents for measuring the pH of tissues. (A) Gd-DOTA-4AMP-F developed by the group of Caravan and colleagues.[35] (B) Gd-L developed by the group of Aime and colleagues.[36] In both cases, the PET/single photon emission computed tomography component is used to calculate the concentration of the contrast agent, making the pH measurement using the MR imaging component possible. (Data from Frullano L, Catana C, Benner T, et al. Bimodal MR-PET agent for quantitative pH imaging. Angew Chem Int Edit 2010;49(13):2382–4; and Gianolio E, Maciocco L, Imperio D, et al. Dual MRI-SPECT agent for pH-mapping. Chem Commun 2011;47(5):1539–41.)

REFERENCES

1. Gupta AK, Gupta M. Synthesis and surface engineering of iron oxide nanoparticles for biomedical applications. Biomaterials 2005;26(18):3995–4021.

2. Laurent S, Forge D, Port M, et al. Magnetic iron oxide nanoparticles: synthesis, stabilization, vectorization, physicochemical characterizations, and biological applications. Chem Rev 2008;108(6): 2064–110.

3. Silva AC, Oliveira TR, Mamani JB, et al. Application of hyperthermia induced by superparamagnetic iron oxide nanoparticles in glioma treatment. Int J Nanomedicine 2011;6:591–603.

4. Caravan P. Strategies for increasing the sensitivity of gadolinium based MRI contrast agents. Chem Soc Rev 2006;35(6):512–23.

5. Basu S, Alavi A. Unparalleled contribution of 18F-FDG PET to medicine over 3 decades. J Nucl Med 2008;49(10):17N–21N, 37N.

6. Joshi NV, Vesey AT, Williams MC, et al. 18F-fluoride positron emission tomography for identification of ruptured and high-risk coronary atherosclerotic plaques: a prospective clinical trial. Lancet 2014; 383(9918):705–13.

7. Holland JP, Divilov V, Bander NH, et al. 89Zr-DFO-J591 for immunoPET of prostate-specific membrane antigen expression in vivo. J Nucl Med 2010;51(8): 1293–300.

8. Fani M, Del Pozzo L, Abiraj K, et al. PET of somatostatin receptor-positive tumors using 64Cu- and 68Ga-somatostatin antagonists: the chelate makes the difference. J Nucl Med 2011;52(7):1110–8.

9. Louie A. Multimodality imaging probes: design and challenges. Chem Rev 2010;110(5):3146–95.

10. de Rosales RT. Potential clinical applications of bimodal PET-MRI or SPECT-MRI agents. J Labelled Comp Radiopharm 2014;57(4):298–303.

11. Makowski MR, Ebersberger U, Nekolla S, et al. In vivo molecular imaging of angiogenesis, targeting alphavbeta3 integrin expression, in a patient after acute myocardial infarction. Eur Heart J 2008; 29(18):2201.

12. Buchbender C, Heusner TA, Lauenstein TC, et al. Oncologic PET/MRI, part 1: tumors of the brain, head and neck, chest, abdomen, and pelvis. J Nucl Med 2012;53(6):928–38.

13. Buchbender C, Heusner TA, Lauenstein TC, et al. Oncologic PET/MRI, part 2: bone tumors, soft-tissue tumors, melanoma, and lymphoma. J Nucl Med 2012;53(8):1244–52.

14. Afshar-Oromieh A, Haberkorn U, Schlemmer HP, et al. Comparison of PET/CT and PET/MRI hybrid systems using a 68Ga-labelled PSMA ligand for the diagnosis of recurrent prostate cancer: initial experience. Eur J Nucl Med Mol Imaging 2014; 41(5):887–97.

15. Judenhofer MS, Wehrl HF, Newport DF, et al. Simultaneous PET-MRI: a new approach for functional and morphological imaging. Nat Med 2008;14(4):459–65.

16. Viel T, Talasila KM, Monfared P, et al. Analysis of the growth dynamics of angiogenesis-dependent and -independent experimental glioblastomas by multimodal small-animal PET and MRI. J Nucl Med 2012;53(7):1135–45.

17. Nahrendorf M, Zhang H, Hembrador S, et al. Nanoparticle PET-CT imaging of macrophages in inflammatory atherosclerosis. Circulation 2008;117(3): 379–87.

18. Jarrett BR, Gustafsson B, Kukis DL, et al. Synthesis of 64Cu-labeled magnetic nanoparticles for multimodal imaging. Bioconjug Chem 2008;19(7): 1496–504.

19. Glaus C, Rossin R, Welch MJ, et al. In vivo evaluation of (64)Cu-labeled magnetic nanoparticles as a dual-modality PET/MR imaging agent. Bioconjug Chem 2010;21(4):715–22.

20. Lee HY, Li Z, Chen K, et al. PET/MRI dual-modality tumor imaging using arginine-glycine-aspartic (RGD)-conjugated radiolabeled iron oxide nanoparticles. J Nucl Med 2008;49(8):1371–9.

21. Xie J, Chen K, Huang J, et al. PET/NIRF/MRI triple functional iron oxide nanoparticles. Biomaterials 2010;31(11):3016–22.

22. Choi JS, Park JC, Nah H, et al. A hybrid nanoparticle probe for dual-modality positron emission tomography and magnetic resonance imaging. Angew Chem Int Ed Engl 2008;47(33):6259–62.

23. Cui X, Belo S, Kruger D, et al. Aluminium hydroxide stabilised MnFe2O4 and Fe3O4 nanoparticles as dual-modality contrasts agent for MRI and PET imaging. Biomaterials 2014;35(22):5840–6.

24. de Rosales RTM, Tavare R, Paul RL, et al. Synthesis of Cu-64(II)-Bis(dithiocarbamatebisphosphonate) and its conjugation with superparamagnetic iron oxide nanoparticles: in vivo evaluation as dual-modality PET-MRI agent. Angew Chem Int Ed Engl 2011;50(24):5509–13.

25. Sandiford L, Phinikaridou A, Protti A, et al. Bisphosphonate-anchored PEGylation and radiolabeling of superparamagnetic iron oxide: long-circulating nanoparticles for in vivo multimodal (T1 MRI-SPECT) imaging. ACS Nano 2013;7(1):500–12.

26. Torres Martin de Rosales R, Tavaré R, Glaria A, et al. (99m)Tc-bisphosphonate-iron oxide nanoparticle conjugates for dual-modality biomedical imaging. Bioconjug Chem 2011;22(3):455–65.

27. Madru R, Kjellman P, Olsson F, et al. Tc-99m-Labeled superparamagnetic iron oxide nanoparticles for multimodality SPECT/MRI of sentinel lymph nodes. J Nucl Med 2012;53(3):459–63.

28. Thorek DL, Ulmert D, Diop NF, et al. Non-invasive mapping of deep-tissue lymph nodes in live animals using a multimodal PET/MRI nanoparticle. Nat Commun 2014;5:3097.

29. Chakravarty R, Valdovinos HF, Chen F, et al. Intrinsically germanium-69-labeled iron oxide nanoparticles: synthesis and in-vivo dual-modality PET/MR imaging. Adv Mater 2014;26(30):5119–23.

30. Freund B, Tromsdorf UI, Bruns OT, et al. A simple and widely applicable method to 59Fe-radiolabel monodisperse superparamagnetic iron oxide nanoparticles for in vivo quantification studies. ACS Nano 2012;6(8):7318–25.

31. Hoffman D. Hybrid PET/MRI nanoparticle development and multi-modal imaging: VCU. 2013. Available at: http://scholarscompass.vcu.edu/etd/3253. Accessed June 2015.

32. Truillet C, Bouziotis P, Tsoukalas C, et al. Ultrasmall particles for Gd-MRI and Ga-PET dual imaging. Contrast Media Mol Imaging 2015;10(4):309–19.

33. Lee J, Lee TS, Ryu J, et al. RGD peptide-conjugated multimodal NaGdF4:Yb3+/Er3+ nanophosphors for upconversion luminescence, MR, and PET imaging of tumor angiogenesis. J Nucl Med 2013;54(1):96–103.

34. Newell K, Franchi A, Pouyssegur J, et al. Studies with glycolysis-deficient cells suggest that production of lactic-acid is not the only cause of tumor acidity. Proc Natl Acad Sci U S A 1993;90(3):1127–31.

35. Frullano L, Catana C, Benner T, et al. Bimodal MR-PET agent for quantitative pH imaging. Angew Chem Int Ed Engl 2010;49(13):2382–4.

36. Gianolio E, Maciocco L, Imperio D, et al. Dual MRI-SPECT agent for pH-mapping. Chem Commun 2011;47(5):1539–41.

MR Imaging–Guided Attenuation Correction of PET Data in PET/MR Imaging

CrossMark

David Izquierdo-Garcia, PhD*, Ciprian Catana, MD, PhD

KEYWORDS

- PET/MR imaging • Attenuation correction • MR-AC • Segmentation • Atlas • Template • Artifacts
- Body truncation

KEY POINTS

- Accurate attenuation correction (AC) is required to avoid biasing PET image quantification.
- PET/magnetic resonance (MR) AC (MR-AC) methods aim to provide accurate AC using the information provided from the PET and/or MR images in combined PET/MR scanners.
- MR-AC methods are divided into segmentation-based, atlas-based, and PET-based approaches, each with its own pros and cons.
- Whole-body imaging remains especially challenging, and further efforts need to concentrate on this area in the future.
- Metallic implants, body truncation, hardware correction, motion, and high intersubject and intra-subject variability for lung density are some of the major challenges that future MR-AC approaches would be required to face.

INTRODUCTION

Attenuation correction (AC) is one of the most important corrections that need to be performed in PET imaging (**Fig. 1**). AC methods aim to account for the photon attenuation along each line of response (LOR). For this purpose, maps of the linear attenuation coefficients (LACs) for all the tissues and materials located in the PET field of view (FoV) are generated or integrals of these values along all the LORs are directly measured. As the procedure for including this information in the reconstruction (ie, performing the actual correction) is similar no matter how these values are obtained, from here on the authors refer to the various attenuation map estimation techniques discussed as AC methods. Recently, in parallel with the development of combined PET/MR imaging scanners, a new class of methods that use the magnetic resonance (MR) information AC (MR-AC) has emerged. This task is not trivial because the MR signal is related to proton density and tissue relaxation times, whereas photon attenuation is linked to the electron density of the body tissues. The growing interest in this research field is reflected by the increasing number of publications reporting novel methods or comparisons between the different approaches (**Fig. 2**). However, the authors should note that even in integrated PET/MR imaging scanners, the PET data could also be used to derive LACs (PET-AC methods) with or without using external devices, such as transmission sources (transmission-based AC [Tx] methods).

This review aims to highlight the state-of-the-art methods for MR-AC. The authors' goal is not to

The authors have nothing to disclose.
Department of Radiology, Athinoula A. Martinos Center for Biomedical Imaging, Massachusetts General Hospital, Harvard Medical School, 149 13th Street, Charlestown 02129, MA, USA
* Corresponding author.
E-mail address: davidizq@nmr.mgh.harvard.edu

PET Clin 11 (2016) 129–149
http://dx.doi.org/10.1016/j.cpet.2015.10.002
1556-8598/16/$ – see front matter © 2016 Elsevier Inc. All rights reserved.

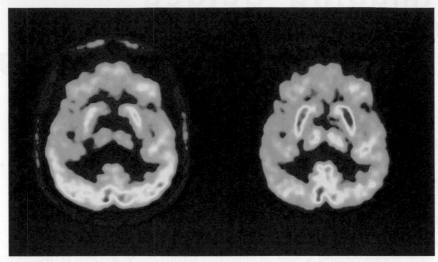

Fig. 1. PET images reconstructed without (*left*) and with (*right*) AC. Note the attenuation effect producing larger reduction of activity toward the center of the head.

provide full methodological details (see references[1,2] for this purpose) but rather to guide the reader through the available alternatives and briefly present their pros and cons. Additionally, the authors discuss those methods that have been proposed for addressing more specific challenges, such as artifacts related to metallic implants, body truncation, and MR hardware. Finally, the authors discuss the latest comparative and clinical studies in which different MR-AC methods have been quantitatively and qualitatively evaluated.

MAGNETIC RESONANCE–ATTENUATION CORRECTION: ATTENUATION CORRECTION METHODS FOR PET/MR IMAGING

Although AC was already known and applied in PET since the early days, the systematic study of AC methods and their effects on PET image quantification started in 1979 with the publication by Huang and colleagues[3] on the "Effects of Inaccurate Attenuation Correction," as part of a series of studies on PET image quantification.[3] This publication was the first to investigate the effects on PET image quantification of inaccurate calculation of the AC factors (ACFs), the mismatch between emission, and transmission and of the noise in ACFs estimation, among others. Since then, several studies have tried to identify solutions to such challenges or to minimize (or eliminate) the need for the time-costly transmission scans.[4,5] More than 35 years later, we are facing similar challenges with a newer technology, PET/MR imaging, such as the need to reduce the errors of MR-AC methods and to minimize the time-consuming data collection required for these approaches (ie, long MR acquisition times).

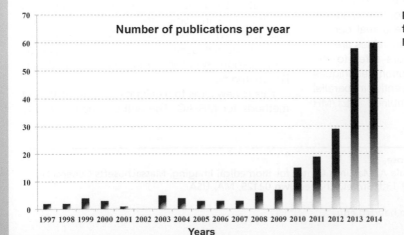

Fig. 2. PubMed results on the following search terms: PET and MR and attenuation correction.

Most of the developed MR-AC methods have focused on brain, and only a handful have been applied to whole-body imaging. This circumstance is because whole-body AC poses more challenges that are more difficult to address appropriately than head AC: higher intersubject anatomic variability, large intrasubject and intersubject lung-density (and therefore attenuation properties) variability, nonrigid motion either due to physiologic (respiratory and cardiac) or nonphysiologic (voluntary) movements, body truncation artifacts, routine use of flexible radiofrequency (RF) coils, difficulty in obtaining MR signal from bone, and so forth. Because of their scarcity, within this review, methods that apply to the whole body are explicitly highlighted in *italics* for an easier identification.

Currently, there are only 3 methods approved by the Food and Drug Administration (FDA) for AC in combined PET/MR imaging: a 3-class (air, soft tissue, and lung) segmentation-based method implemented in the sequential Philips PET/MR scanner[6,7] and two 4-class (air, fat, soft tissue, and lungs) segmentation-based methods implemented in the simultaneous Siemens scanner that was based on the work of Martinez-Moller and colleagues[8] and in the new simultaneous time-of-flight (ToF) PET/MR from GE for whole-body imaging.[9] None of them properly accounts for bone tissue attenuation, which has been shown to produce large PET image bias (**Fig. 3**). Additionally, the GE approach also uses an atlas approach

for head AC that does include bone tissue as a separate class. A myriad of MR-AC methods have recently been proposed and compared with the commercially available ones. These methods can be grouped into 3 main categories: 2 MR-based (segmentation- and atlas-based methods) and one emission-based method (PET-AC) that includes joint estimation, emission-based-only methods, and Tx-AC approaches.

Segmentation-Based Methods

Rationale
Segmentation-based methods rely on the accurate segmentation (classification) of MR images into separate attenuating tissue classes. Once segmented, a unique LAC is assigned to each tissue class. The segmentation/classification step is critical to obtain optimal results, in addition to the appropriate choice of the LAC for each tissue class. Although this review intentionally does not discuss here the effect of the LAC choice, this issue has been addressed in other reviews (eg, see references[1,2]).

Challenges, pros, and cons
The main challenges for MR-based segmentation-based methods are twofold. First, the accurate and robust segmentation of various tissue classes becomes even more challenging in the case of MR because the lack of absolute quantification of the MR imaging signal makes the translation of the

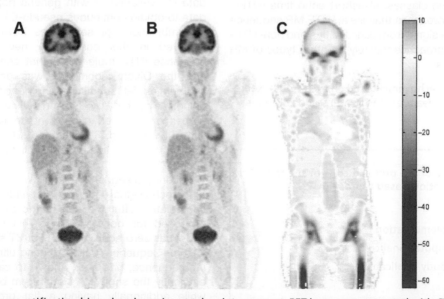

Fig. 3. Image quantification bias when bone is not taken into account: PET image reconstructed with CT-AC (*A*) or with the same CT-AC but with all bone structures set to the attenuation value of soft tissue (*B*) and relative differences in percentage (*C*). (*From* Hofmann M, Pichler B, Schölkopf B, et al. Towards quantitative PET/MRI: a review of MR-based attenuation correction techniques. Eur J Nucl Med Mol Imaging 2009;36(Suppl 1):S101; with permission.)

algorithms more difficult and the nonhomogeneity of the main magnetic field leads to image intensity bias. Second, the small (and often null) signal obtained with standard MR sequences from bone tissues due to its very rapid T2* relaxation times complicates its segmentation from the air cavities (also with very low or null MR signal). Accurate air and bone segmentation is critical because they are the extremes in terms of LACs, 0 cm^{-1} for air and 0.150 cm^{-1} and greater for cortical bone.[10]

The pros and cons of the segmentation-based MR-AC methods are summarized in **Box 1**.

First steps

The first MR segmentation method was reported in 1994. It focused on the brain and used a surface registration algorithm to align the MR (a T1-weighted image) with the PET image.[11] Once in the same space, the MR images were segmented using morphologic operations combined with hard thresholds to obtain brain, skull, and skin. LACs were finally assigned to each tissue class: 0.095 cm^{-1} to brain and skin and 0.151 cm^{-1} to bone. Almost a decade later, an improved approach was proposed in which the coregistered MR (also a T1-weighted image) was segmented, via a fuzzy clustering algorithm, into 4 classes: air, skull, brain tissue, and nasal sinuses.[12]

State of the art

Since 2009, several proposed methods generated promising results. These methods can be grouped into 2 main classes: ultrashort echo time (UTE)–based approaches that use an UTE MR sequence to provide signal from bone tissues and non–UTE-based approaches that rely on other types of MR sequences.

Ultrashort echo time–based In 2010, both Keereman and colleagues[13] and Catana and colleagues[14]

independently used for the first time a UTE sequence to obtain signal from bone tissue, which helped with its segmentation from the rest of the tissue classes. Catana and colleagues[14] used the difference of the two echoes divided by the second echo squared to enhance bone voxels and the sum of the two echoes divided by the first echo squared to enhance voxels corresponding to air (**Fig. 4**). Keereman and colleagues[13] used the inverse of the spin-spin relaxation time T2, called relaxation rate (or simply R2), to segment bone from the other tissue classes. The R2 was defined as the difference of the logarithmic echo images over the difference of the echo times. In a modified version of this approach, the magnetic field was dynamically monitored by using a magnetic field camera, which allowed the correction of the k-space trajectory distortions induced by the eddy currents artifacts.[15] A new Dixon-based strategy to obtain relaxation rates (R2*) from UTE sequences was used in a study by Hu and colleagues.[16] Interestingly, the investigators also explored and optimized the k-space sampling to reduce the acquisition time by 75%, while preserving the image quality and contrast in cortical bone.

Two different methods to convert the relaxation times R2* into continuous computed tomography (CT) values have recently been explored. The first used a regression analysis to map the R2* values into pseudo-CT values via a 5-parameter sigmoid function.[17] In the second approach, the R2* data was equalized with either patient-specific CT data (if available) or with generic population CT data to obtain continuous pseudo-CT values.[18]

Combinations of sequences have also been explored in this context. A new triple-echo sequence (UTE triple echo) that combined UTE and the Dixon techniques was developed to segment air, fat, soft tissue, and bone for brain imaging.[19] In a study by Hsu and colleagues,[20] fuzzy C-means were used to segment the data acquired with T1-weighted, T2-weighted, UTE, ToF, and Dixon sequences to segment skull, fat, soft tissue, and air.

Recently, a sequence that allows the acquisition of the echo signal (known as free induction decay) immediately after the end of the excitation was proposed for bone imaging. This sequence is known as zero echo time (ZT) or ZT sequence. A ZT-type sequence, called rotating ultrafast imaging sequence, has been shown to capture more efficiently the short T2* signal from bone tissues while additionally having a flat proton-density response in soft tissues.[21] A clinical evaluation of the use of ZT sequence has also been recently performed in 15 subjects[22] showing great potential to produce CT-like images (**Fig. 5**).

Box 1
Summary of the pros and cons of the MR-AC segmentation-based approaches

Pros

Easy implementation

Low computational cost

Whole-body applicability

Cons

Robustness (noise, bias)

Bone/air segmentation

Discrete LACs

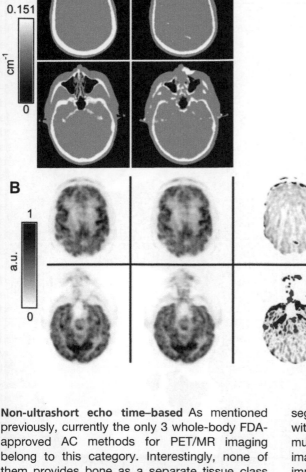

Fig. 4. Use of UTE sequence for MR-AC application: (*A*) μ-maps for segmented CT-AC (*left*) and UTE-based MR-AC (*right*). (*B*) Reconstructed PET images using CT-AC (*left*) and UTE-based MR-AC (*middle*) and their relative differences (*right*). a.u., arbitrary units; RC, relative change. (This research was originally published in *JNM*. Catana C, van der Kouwe A, Benner T, et al. Toward implementing an MRI-based PET attenuation-correction method for neurologic studies on the MR-PET brain prototype. J Nucl Med 2010;51(9):1436. © by the Society of Nuclear Medicine and Molecular Imaging, Inc.)

Non-ultrashort echo time–based As mentioned previously, currently the only 3 whole-body FDA-approved AC methods for PET/MR imaging belong to this category. Interestingly, none of them provides bone as a separate tissue class but are applied to brain and *whole-body* imaging, except in the case of the GE approach that uses an atlas for brain images. The first one uses a Vibe Dixon sequence with in-phase and out-of-phase images to separate fat-based from water-based tissues.[8] This Dixon-based method produces an attenuation map with 4 tissue classes: air, soft tissue, fat, and lungs, with the lungs obtained as the connected air class inside the body. The AC approach was based on this method.[2] A similar approach is followed for whole body on the GE PET/MR scanner using the Dixon sequence to provide continuous fat/water AC values, lung, and air.[9] The third one, implemented on the Philips scanner, classified a T1-weighted image into 3 tissues: soft tissue, air, or lungs.[6,7] A similar 3-class segmentation approach was also tested on beagles using T1-weighted images and compared with a 4-class approach including bone from a registered CT.[23]

The use of fuzzy classifiers has recurrently been proposed for segmentation. A minimal path segmentation approach (similar to segmentation with snakes) was implemented followed by a multi-scale fuzzy C-mean classifier for brain images.[24] This approach was subsequently improved by including a radon transform of the MR image (T1 weighted) to segment the skull from the brain.[25,26]

Take home comparative results

Fig. 6 shows a comparative plot of the MR-AC segmentation-based methods. Only data available in the original articles are included. Despite the authors' efforts to include comparable values in this plot, as well as in **Figs. 9** and **12**, care must be taken when comparing them because the methodology followed varied from study to study.

Atlas-Based Methods

Rationale

Atlas-based methods use a dataset (or multiple datasets) for which the LACs are known or could be derived from (eg, CT images). The dataset is then mapped into the subject specific MR space, either via nonrigid coregistration (using the atlas as a template) or via probabilistic methods. Although not necessarily, in most cases, the atlases are composed of pairs of image datasets:

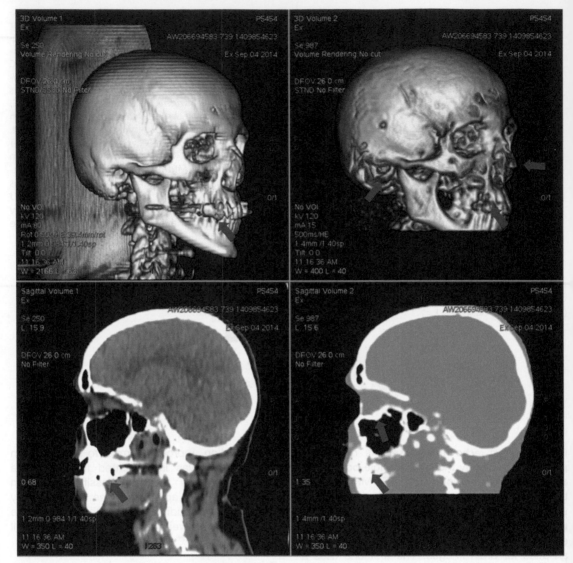

Fig. 5. Segmentation results obtained with a ZT sequence (*right*) and its comparison with a CT image (*left*). Arrows point to dental artifacts, minor misclassification of cartilage and auditory canal air, and oversegmentation on the sinuses. (This research was originally published in *JNM*. Delso G, Wiesinger F, Sacolick LI, et al. Clinical evaluation of zero-echo-time MR imaging for the segmentation of the skull. J Nucl Med 2015;56(3):419. © by the Society of Nuclear Medicine and Molecular Imaging, Inc.)

the atlas MR image (generated from data acquired with a similar MR sequence to the one to be used for the new subjects) and the atlas image with the LACs information (ie, transmission or CT images).

Challenges, pros, and cons

The major challenge for atlas-based methods is the difficulty in warping local anatomic variants, particularly for the whole-body case. However, atlas-based methods provide bone information and continuous attenuation values that tend to improve the final PET image quantification when compared with segmented approaches. A

summary of the pros and cons of the atlas-based MR-AC approaches is shown in **Box 2**.

First steps

The first atlas-based method used the well-known Statistical Parametric Mapping, University College London (SPM2) to spatially normalize the PET image of the subject to the PET image of an atlas and the corresponding atlas transmission image.[27] The transmission image was then warped back into the (PET) subject space using the inverse deformations estimated during the spatial normalization process. As a result, a subject-specific

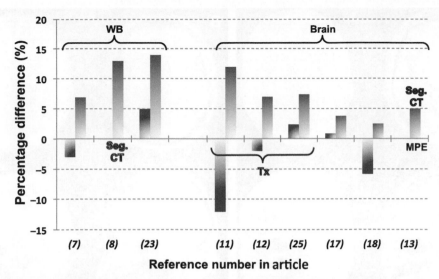

Fig. 6. Comparison of minimum (*red*) and maximum (*blue*) percentage differences of PET reconstructed images versus the gold standard, CT-AC, unless explicitly written otherwise. Where available, mean percentage error (MPE) replaces maximum percentage differences. Seg CT, segmented CT AC. (*Data from* Refs.[7,8,11–13,17,18,23,25])

transmission image is generated in subject (PET) space. A similar strategy using SPM2 was used to spatially normalize the subject images to an atlas composed of transmission images and T1-weighted MR images (instead of the PET images as in the previous case).[28] Both studies showed comparable results, the mean differences in the brain being approximately 10%.

State of the art

Atlas-based methods could be further classified into 2 main groups: the template-based approaches, whereby the template images are non-rigidly warped back into the subject space (like in the first methods), and probabilistic-based approaches, whereby the atlas information is used via probabilistic or machine learning techniques to generate a pseudo-CT image. Additionally, a third group could be defined as the mixed-based

Box 2
Summary of the pros and cons of the atlas-based MR-AC approaches
Pros
Robustness (noise, bias)
Bone identification
Continuous LACs
Cons
Subject-specific variability
Whole-body
Computational cost

approaches that include those methods combining elements from the first two approaches.

Template based In this group we find the first method specifically implemented for *whole-body* applications (besides the two segmentation-based methods presented earlier). The approach used a nonrigid algorithm to register the atlas CT images to the subject MR image and a histogram-matching algorithm to map MR values into final pseudo-CT values.[29] The method was tested for head and neck, thoracic, abdominal and pelvic imaging with errors larger than 10% in some regions.

A nonrigid algorithm based on optical flow was used to coregister the template CT to the subject MR image in Schreibmann and colleagues.[30] Although the investigators showed excellent agreement between the CT and pseudo-CT images obtained (with a mean difference in all voxels of 2 Hounsfield units), only data from a single PET study was shown and no figures of merit (such as relative differences or similar) were given. Malone and colleagues[31] compared the SPM2 and B-splines nonrigid algorithms for coregistration of the atlas MR images into the subject MR, using either a tissue phantom or a transmission template as atlas pairs together with the MRs (**Fig. 7**). The investigators concluded based on the analysis of reconstructed PET brain images that the transmission template approach was better than the tissue phantom and that B-splines was better than SPM2.[31] In a different approach, an atlas was composed of 121 CT scans and weighted heuristic measures were used to choose the most similar CT to the subject's MR in terms of body geometry, which was nonrigidly

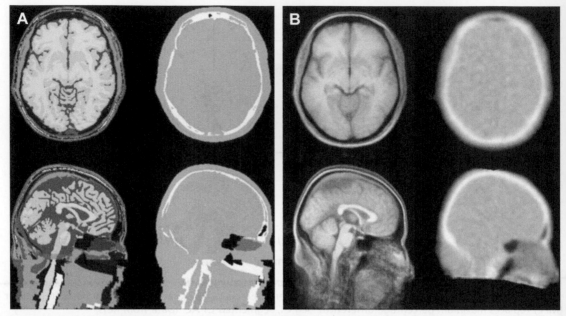

Fig. 7. Axial (*top row*) and sagittal (*bottom row*) slices for MR imaging and attenuation maps for a tissue atlas (*A*) and a template created using VTK CISG (Visualization Toolkit, Computational Imaging Sciences Group, King's College London) (*B*). (This research was originally published in *JNM*. Malone IB, Ansorge RE, Williams GB, et al. Attenuation correction methods suitable for brain imaging with a PET/MRI scanner: a comparison of tissue atlas and template attenuation map approaches. J Nucl Med 2011;52(7):1144. © by the Society of Nuclear Medicine and Molecular Imaging, Inc.)

coregistered to the subject's MR.[32] Two segmentation-based methods were generated and compared: the standard 4-tissue segmentation (air, fat, soft tissue, and lung) and a second one that included additionally the bone derived from the warped atlas CT image. The comparisons showed that the method including the atlas-CT bone reduced the errors in bone and adjacent regions of interest (ROIs); however, the "correlation coefficient was essentially unchanged in all tissues regardless of whether bone was included or not."[32]

A brain atlas-based approach combining nonrigid coregistration plus similarity measurements was used to generate a pseudo-CT image.[33,34] The technique nonrigidly registers the atlas MR images into the subject MR image (all MRs are T1-weighted images) and uses the resulting deformations to warp the atlas CTs into subject space. Instead of using an average of all the warped CTs, the approach calculates similarities between each warped MR atlas image and the original subject image by using a convolution-based fast local normalized correlation coefficient similarity measure. The final pseudo-CT image is generated by a linear combination of all atlas-CT images weighted by an exponential function of the ranked similarities.[33] The method was optimized using 18 subjects, and then it was successfully tested on another 41 subjects using the

subject PET reconstructed with CT-AC as the gold standard and comparing the results with a UTE-based segmentation method (air, soft tissue, and bone) as well as to the best warped CT image from the atlas.[34] As a way to obtain warped CT images closer to the subject space, an iterative scheme was chosen to recoregister the warped atlas CTs to their mean until convergence. Finally, a median filter was applied to obtain the final pseudo-CT from all the warped CTs.[35]

Probabilistic based The use of probabilistic and machine learning techniques has grown in the recent years because of their potential to benefit whole-body applications and the quality of their results. A gaussian mixture regression (GMR) approach was used to generate pseudo-CT images from the subject MR images.[36] The atlas images consisted of 1 CT image and 15 MR images per subject, consisting of 3 versions (original, mean, and standard deviation images) of the images acquired with each of the following 5 MR sequences: the two echoes of two different UTE acquisitions (with different flip angles) and one T2-weighted sequence. For any new subject, the same 5 MR images (generating the 15 MR datasets) were acquired and the regression model was applied to then generate a pseudo-CT image.[36] In later studies the investigators found that the T2-weighted sequence was redundant in terms of the information provided and, therefore, was dropped from the regression model.[37] A comparative study of the resulting PET images showed results comparable with those obtained using the real CTs.[38] Additional improvements have been demonstrated by adding spatial information[39] as well by reducing the acquisition time for the UTE sequences with parallel imaging.[40] A similar approach but using support vector regression (SVR) machinery instead of GMR was used to model the mapping between the atlas CT and MR images (using a UTE and a Dixon sequence, with image features extracted for mean, median, variance, maximum, and minimum).[41] Once trained, the SVR machinery was applied to predict a pseudo-CT image from the subject MR images. Although the investigators mostly focused on the brain with great results, the method was also used to generate the attenuation map of the pelvis for one subject, which suggests it could be used for *whole-body* imaging as well.[41]

Despite their high computational cost, patch-based methods have recently received renewed attention because of their robustness and potential adaptability to whole-body applications. They use local probabilistic and similarity measures to compare a region (known as patch) of the subject's MR image with the whole MR database. The best patch (or patches) from the atlas database that fits the subject is chosen and its corresponding CT patch is used to obtain a pseudo-CT image. The first implementation of a patch-based approach combined it with a nonrigid registration to an atlas and a classic segmentation-based method.[42] The method was initially tested for brain imaging but subsequently applied to *whole-body* imaging, showing results superior to the segmentation-based method with 5 classes (lung, bone, fat, soft tissue, and a mixture of fat and soft tissue).[43] Others have also proposed pure patch-based approaches for brain imaging, either using T1-weighted images combined with probabilistic air maps to separate bone and air[44] or the two UTE echoes as atlases in addition to a gaussian mixture model (GMM) to provide all convex linear combinations of pairs of atlases to reduce the sparsity problem linked to patch-based methods.[45] To address the large computational cost, a GPU (graphics processing unit) based algorithm based on a weighted linear combination of the atlas CT images with weights based on their similarity was proposed.[46]

Mixed based An atlas-guided segmentation technique has demonstrated improved results when compared with the original UTE based only approach for brain imaging.[47] More recently, it has been shown that a combination of segmentation- and atlas-based features confers flexibility to adapt to the local anatomic variants of the subject (thanks to the segmentation step) and robustness thanks to the nonrigid diffeomorphic registration to a template.[48] This approach, developed using the SPM8 software for both the image segmentation and nonrigid coregistration steps, generated very good results using datasets acquired at different institutions (**Fig. 8**).[48] Similarly, Anazodo and colleagues[49] used an SPM8-based approach to combine the Dixon-based method with the bone segmentation generated from SPM8.

Take home comparative results
Fig. 9 shows a comparative plot of the MR-AC atlas-based methods.

PET–Attenuation Correction

Rationale
PET-AC methods aim at using the emission PET data that inherently contain information about the attenuation or derive the LACs. Therefore, these methods are well suited for whole-body applications, although in most cases they require a nonspecific radiotracer to provide information for all tissues. There are 3 main classes of PET-AC methods: approaches that derive attenuation maps by postprocessing the emission images (emission based); approaches that aim to jointly estimate emission and attenuation (joint estimation based methods) using iterative algorithms based on maximum likelihood (ML); and approaches that use external transmission sources to derive the LACs (Tx based). Because no MR images are required (in principle) for the PET-AC methods, approaches in this category were developed earlier compared with the other MR-AC methods, to be used in stand-alone PET (and PET/CT) scanners.

Challenges, pros, and cons
Until recently, postprocessing the emission data allowed only the approximate estimation of the actual LACs (segmented AC maps). Deriving emission and attenuation images jointly from the PET raw data is a very ill-posed problem that results in crosstalk between both estimations.[50–52] Crosstalk is characterized by the presence of localized errors in the emission map, which are compensated by errors in the attenuation map. Solving the crosstalk problem requires additional information, either a priori (from MR or other imaging modality) or ToF information. Joint estimation also requires that sufficient counts are recorded in all the lines of response that intersect the attenuation map. Finally, the Tx-based approaches,

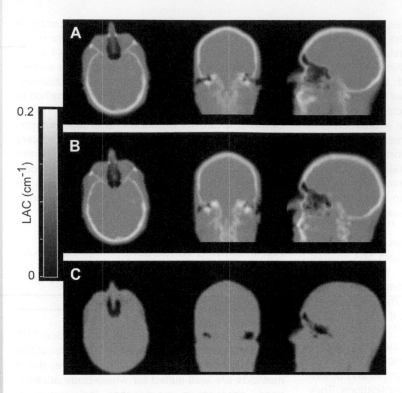

Fig. 8. Comparison of attenuation maps from new SPM8 atlas method (*A*), from CT (*B*), and from Dixon-based method (*C*). (This research was originally published in *JNM*. An SPM8-based approach for attenuation correction combining segmentation and nonrigid template formation: application to simultaneous PET/MR brain imaging. J Nucl Med 2014;55(11):1826. © by the Society of Nuclear Medicine and Molecular Imaging, Inc.)

considered the real gold standard for AC in PET as they measure the attenuation at PET energy levels (and are more immune to metal artifacts), involve additional radiation exposure to the subject (although minimal compared with PET or CT scans), an extended acquisition time (unless the transmission and emission data are collected simultaneously), and an increase in detector dead time and tend to produce more noisy estimations of the LACs. A summary of the pros and cons of the PET-AC approaches is shown in **Box 3**.

First steps

Because PET-AC methods were developed for stand-alone PET scanners, the first Tx-based approach was reported in 1975 and used a ring

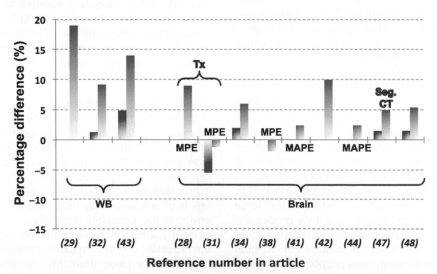

Fig. 9. Comparison of minimum (*red*) and maximum (*blue*) percentage differences of PET reconstructed images versus the gold standard, CT-AC, unless explicitly written otherwise. Where available, mean percentage error (MPE) or mean absolute percentage error (MAPE) replaces maximum percentage differences. Seg CT, segmented CT-AC; WB, whole body. (*Data from* Refs.[28,29,31,32,34,38,41–44,47,48])

Box 3
Summary of the pros and cons of the PET-AC approaches

Pros

MR time for clinical use

Robust to artifacts

Implants body truncation, hardware attenuation

Whole-body applicability

Cons

Crosstalk and emission data in all LORs (joint based)

Computational cost (joint based)

Extended acquisition time (Tx)

Noise + additional radiation (Tx)

Accuracy (emission based)

of Copper-64 positioned around the subject (a dog in this case).[53] The first joint-based algorithm was also developed before the first PET/MR was introduced and used an ML estimator with an expectation-maximization scheme.[50] The method applied kernel sieves to constrain the solution and minimize its bias.

State of the art

Emission based Before PET/MR scanners, emission-based approaches were developed to either reduce the noise and variability of the transmission images or completely replace the transmission scans to reduce both the radiation exposure and acquisition times. In an early method, simple segmented attenuation maps were obtained from the emission data using the sinogram information.[54] The same information was also used to segment and estimate the LACs for the skull and the rest of the brain.[5] More recently a 3-step PET reconstruction process was used to segment lungs and body contour from the intermediate PET reconstructed images.[55]

Finally, the scatter information has been proposed to derive LACs using a 2-level approach: a scatter-to-attenuation reconstructor and a scatter-to-attenuation back projector.[56] Although the method is still in its initial development phase and comes with an extremely large computational cost, very interesting and promising results have been demonstrated with simulated data.

Joint estimation based The joint estimation of transmission and emission images was first demonstrated using an ML algorithm.[57] In a similar approach, the simultaneous estimation was performed after the two images were initially estimated separately.[58] Nuyts and colleagues[51] extended the use of simultaneous joint estimation without the need of transmission images, in an approach called ML reconstruction of attenuation and activity (MLAA). ToF information was incorporated subsequently in Salomon and colleagues[59] and Rezaei and colleagues[60] to reduce the crosstalk, although this was shown to determine the attenuation map sinogram (for all lines of response where activity is present) only up to a constant factor.[61] This constant factor can be determined by imposing an a priori knowledge of the attenuation value in a portion of the attenuation map. A recently developed method using GMM in addition to ToF information[62] was shown to be superior to the standard 4-class MR-AC (**Fig. 10**) as well as to the standard MLAA methods discussed earlier.[63]

Tx based Finally, the use of transmission sources seems to be having its second youth with PET/MR imaging. The use of an annulus transmission source combined with the ToF information was demonstrated in Mollet and colleagues[64] and 2 years later was applied to real PET studies in humans (**Fig. 11**).[65] A single ring transmission source and a multi-bed transmission-emission strategy was recently proposed for non–ToF-capable PET/MR scanners.[66] An interesting alternative uses the background radiation of the lutetium oxyorthosilicate (LSO) scintillators to simultaneously acquire emission and transmission images using different energy windows and the ToF information.[67]

Take home comparative results
Fig. 12 shows a comparative plot of the PET-AC methods.

MAGNETIC RESONANCE–ATTENUATION CORRECTION: SOURCES OF ARTIFACTS AND OTHER CHALLENGES

In addition to accurately translating the MR information into precise LACs, the MR-AC methods need to minimize the potential impact of artifacts in the PET/MR images that could bias the estimation of the LACs. For example, artifacts caused by metallic implants within the MR FoV or truncation due to limited MR FoV need to be considered (**Fig. 13**). Additionally, the attenuation of hardware components present in the FoV of the PET/MR scanner, such as MR RF coils and other equipment (headphones, positioning aids, and so forth), has to be accounted for.

A very challenging region for whole-body AC is the thorax because the lung tissue exhibits large intrasubject and intersubject density variability[68,69] and only a handful of studies have

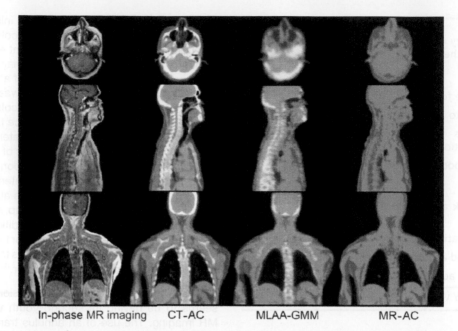

In-phase MR imaging   CT-AC   MLAA-GMM   MR-AC

Fig. 10. Comparison of μ-maps using MLAA-GMM method, the standard 4-class segment MR-AC method, and their reference CT-AC. (This research was originally published in *JNM*. Mehranian A, Zaidi H. Clinical assessment of emission- and segmentation-based MRI-guided attenuation correction in whole-body TOF PET/MRI. J Nucl Med 2015;56(6):879. © by the Society of Nuclear Medicine and Molecular Imaging, Inc.)

tackled this problem. A method to relate the MR imaging and CT signals from the lungs was developed in Marshall and colleagues.[70] Pulmonary lesions were evaluated with the Dixon-method in Jena and colleagues,[71] and the use of PET/MR in lung cancer was examined in Yoon and colleagues.[72] Additionally, motion impacts the accuracy of AC methods and is even more critical in whole-body imaging because of the combination of physiologic and nonphysiologic subject motion. Motion correction in PET/MR is a separate very active area of research, and the authors refer the interested reader to a dedicated review focused on challenges and potential solutions.[73]

This section reviews the latest approaches to address these issues. The authors have grouped them into 3 main categories: body-truncation correction, foreign object correction (such as

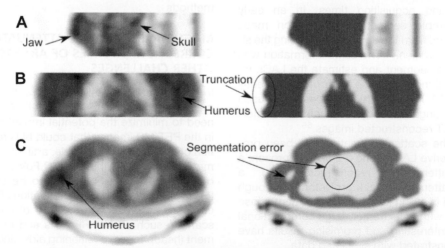

Fig. 11. Comparison of transmission-based (*left*) versus segmentation-based MR-AC (*right*) on 3 subjects: for head and neck (*A*), torso in coronal view (*B*), and torso in axial view (*C*). (This research was originally published in *JNM*. Mollet P, Keereman V, Bini J, et al. Improvement of attenuation correction in time-of-flight PET/MR imaging with a positron-emitting source. J Nucl Med 2014;55(2):334. © by the Society of Nuclear Medicine and Molecular Imaging, Inc.)

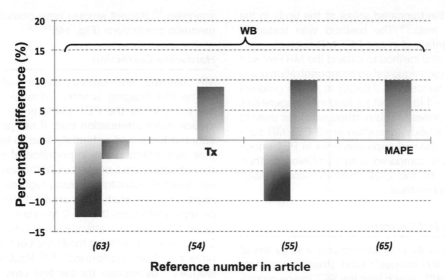

Fig. 12. Comparison of minimum (*red*) and maximum (*blue*) percentage differences of PET reconstructed images versus the gold standard, CT-AC, unless explicitly written otherwise. Where available, mean absolute percentage error (MAPE) replaces maximum percentage differences. (*Data from* Refs.[54,55,63,65])

metallic implants), and hardware correction (such as MR flexible coils).

Body-Truncation Correction

Body-truncation artifacts occur because of the limited effective FoV of the MR imaging compared with that of the PET scanner. In the case of relatively large patients, the MR images may not include the whole patients anatomy, which impacts the performance of the MR-AC approaches. It has been shown that the bias introduced by incomplete attenuation maps is on average 15% but could locally reach up to

50%.[74] A truncation-correction method was proposed for segmenting the body contour with a 3D snake algorithm from the PET images reconstructed with incomplete attenuation information. Even with this method, local errors of up to 20% were still obtained near the edge of the MR FoV. A similar method used the PET data reconstructed with incomplete attenuation information to obtain the body contour of the subject and was compared with the manufacturer's algorithm that obtained the body contour from the PET nonattenuation corrected (NAC) image.[75] A maximum-a-posteriori (MAP) algorithm was included as a modification of the original MLAA approach for

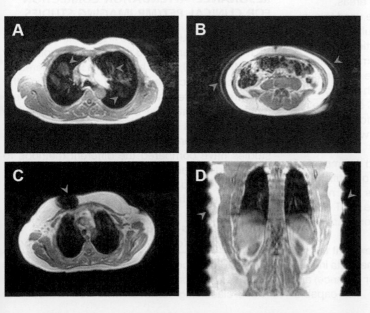

Fig. 13. Examples of common MR artifacts (*arrowheads*) that impact the quality of MR-AC approaches: flow (*A*) and respiratory motion artifacts (*B*), metallic implant (*C*), and body truncation artifacts due to limited FoV (*D*). (*From* Izquierdo-Garcia D, Sawiak SJ, Knesaurek K, et al. Comparison of MR-based attenuation correction and CT-based attenuation correction of whole-body PET/MR imaging. Eur J Nucl Med Mol Imaging 2014;41(8):1582; with permission.)

estimating the truncated areas of the body in the attenuation map.[76] The method was tested in simulated data and in one PET/MR subject.

Finally, a new method to extend the MR FoV was based on a technique called homogenization using gradient enhancement (HUGE) in which gradient fields are used to correct for field inhomogeneities and nonlinearities.[77] This method was later used to minimize the body truncation in 12 PET/MR subjects[78] and showed improvements in PET image quantification compared with the Dixon method as well as to the previously mentioned MAP MLAA-based method.

Foreign Object Correction

Metallic implants tend to produce a large signal void in the MR images[79] (and streaking artifacts in CT images[80]), which bias the PET image quantification when MR-AC methods are used.

Three alternatives to the original Dixon method were suggested to correct for the effect of MR artifacts due to metallic implants in the pelvic area. The first was to fill the signal void with soft tissue. In the second case, a coregistered CT attenuation map of the implant was superimposed on the map generated earlier. In the third case, the signal void was filled with metal.[81] Not surprisingly, the conclusion was that the second approach was the best. A modified version of the patch-based method shown in Hofmann and colleagues[43] added an extra class to include low MR signal regions (due to either air pockets inside the gastrointestinal tract or metallic implants).[82] Separation of air pockets and metallic implant areas was then performed via an atlas that provided a priori information of probable metallic implant areas.

Newer MR sequences can also be used to minimize the extent of the artifacts. A multi-acquisition variable resonance image combination (MAVRIC) MR sequence was used to reduce metal artifacts from dental implants and improve the performance of the MR-AC when compared with the conventional Dixon method.[83] The MAVRIC sequence requires long acquisition times; therefore, its use is only justified in very specific areas where the implants are located.

Lois and colleagues[84] also studied the impact of MR contrast agents on PET image quantification. They concluded that these agents are not expected to significantly impact the PET image quantification, but oral iron-oxide contrasts might bias the MR-AC maps.

It is worth mentioning in this context that the effects of image artifacts as well as other data inconsistencies (in the attenuation map for instance) are supposed to be reduced in ToF-capable scanners.[85] Recent studies have confirmed these theoretic predictions (**Fig. 14**).[86-88]

Hardware Correction

MR coils and other devices are generally invisible to the MR imaging scanner. However, they are not invisible to the PET photons and generally induce extra attenuation that, if not properly accounted for, could potentially lead to large image bias and artifacts. The importance of accounting for the attenuation properties of the MR hardware has been demonstrated using high-exposure CT images.[89] The study also showed that accurate coregistration (less than 1–2 mm) is mandatory to avoid important attenuation-driven artifacts. Similar studies showing the impact of surface coils have also been performed.[90-92] Paulus and colleagues[93] developed for the first time a method to correct for MR surface coils. They used MR visible markers (cod liver oil capsules) positioned on top of the coils to allow for accurate nonrigid registration of the coil to its CT-derived template.[93] The same investigators also provided an improved conversion of the CT image of the coil template to LACs at PET energy levels (511 keV).[94] A similar nonrigid coregistration of the flexible coils to its attenuation template has been suggested in Kartmann and colleagues.[95]

Finally, certain positioning aids, such as vacuum mattresses, were also shown to bias the PET images.[96] Similarly, the use of headphones in PET/MR studies could result in an underestimation in local areas from 1.9% to 13.2%.[97]

CURRENT STATUS OF MAGNETIC RESONANCE–ATTENUATION CORRECTION FOR CLINICAL PET/MR IMAGING STUDIES

Since the introduction of the first human combined PET/MR scanner in 2008 and the first whole-body PET/MR in 2010, there has been a lot of interest in addressing the challenges and demonstrating the benefits of this technology. Recognizing the qualitative and quantitative effects of MR-AC on the PET images has led to the myriad of methods that are reviewed here. Additionally, a large number of studies have compared the different methods to better understand their benefits and/or limitations. Finally, more and more clinical evaluation and comparison studies have also been carried out.

Clinical Studies Evaluating Magnetic Resonance–Attenuation Correction Methods

The need to account for bone in MR-AC methods has been demonstrated in several studies.[98-101] The 3-class segmentation MR-AC method was

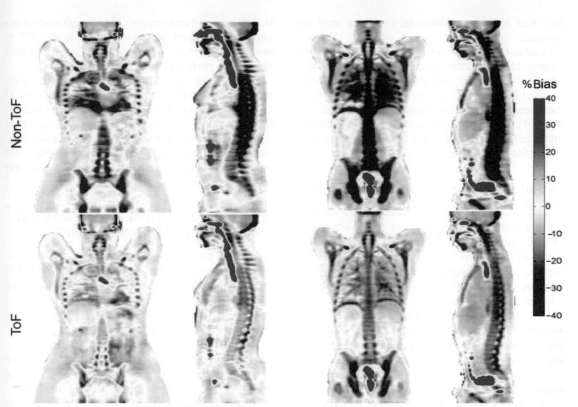

Fig. 14. Comparison of bias between the standard 4-class segmentation MR-AC approach and CT-AC with non-ToF (*top row*) and ToF (*bottom row*) capabilities. (This research was originally published in *JNM*. Mehranian A, Zaidi H. Impact of time-of-flight PET on quantification errors in MR imaging-based attenuation correction. J Nucl Med 2015;56(4):636. © by the Society of Nuclear Medicine and Molecular Imaging, Inc.)

compared with the transmission-based AC in Schramm and colleagues[102] and to the CT-AC in Partovi and colleagues[103] and Izquierdo-Garcia and colleagues.[69] This last study compared the MR-AC methods in 2 groups, with and without the MR coils in the FoV, as well as performing a clinical evaluation and comparison of all PET reconstructed images, including the frequency and effects of artifacts in the attenuation map and the PET reconstructed images.[69] The investigators concluded that the presence of the coils in the FoV increases the variability in PET image quantification and that MR-AC compared with CT-AC introduces a bias of around 10% in whole body, with some ROIs showing larger differences (eg, spine, lung, and heart). The same comparison with CT-AC was also performed in a preclinical model and showed comparable results.[104]

Andersen and colleagues[105] compared the Dixon method (4-class segmentation) implemented on the Siemens PET/MR scanner to the CT-AC method for brain imaging, demonstrating once again the need to include bone to avoid large radial biases across the brain. A whole-body comparison of the Dixon-based with the CT-AC method

was also performed in Aznar and colleagues[106] showing large bias in individual subjects (of up to 22%), which according to the investigators "is significant during clinical follow-up exams."[106] A study of the impact of artifacts on the Dixon-based method was performed retrospectively on 100 PET/MR patients with 276 artifacts.[107] The study showed that 21% of the avid-PET lesions detected were affected by artifacts, mostly without clinical consequences except in 9 lesions that could have been missed because of the artifacts. The investigators clarified that the combined use of the PET-NAC or additional MR images helped with the detection of these lesions so the biased maps would not affect the clinical diagnosis.[107]

A comparison of the Dixon- and UTE-based methods (also implemented on the Siemens PET/MR scanner[13]) versus CT-AC was done for brain imaging in Dickson and colleagues.[108] The investigators showed large underestimations with both methods, Dixon and UTE based, when compared with CT-AC. Delso and colleagues[109] also compared the same UTE-based method versus CT-AC for brain imaging and concluded that in some areas the UTE-method led to bias and that more sophisticated methods may be needed.

Finally, the performance of the Philips 3-class segmentation and the Siemens 4-class segmentation method were compared with the CT-AC. Large biases were observed for both MR-AC methods, and the investigators suggested the need of checking the attenuation map for potential artifacts that could bias the standardized uptake value (SUV) measurements.[110]

Clinical Studies Highlighting the Importance of Accurate Attenuation Correction

Clinical evaluation of the impact of artifacts in the MR-AC has been performed in several studies, such as the previously mentioned Izquierdo-Garcia and colleagues[69] and Arabi and colleagues[110] but also in Keller and colleagues[111] whereby similar conclusions were drawn: the use of PET-AC together with PET-NAC and other MR images improves the detection of artifact-driven bias in the images and "ensure clinically accurate image interpretation."

The Dixon method has been clinically evaluated in multiple occasions. In the early studies, it was shown to be valid for "anatomic allocation of PET-positive lesions, similar to low-dose CT in conventional PET/CT"[112] as well as for oncologic studies.[113] Fraum and colleagues[114] discussed MR-AC in the context of abdominal and pelvic oncological PET/MR use, whereas Schafer and colleagues[115] compared MR-AC and CT-AC in pediatric oncological subjects. The investigators concluded that SUV quantification was similar and the rates of lesion detection were equivalent, with the advantage of the lower radiation exposure from the PET/MR.[115] The Dixon method in PET/MR was also compared with contrast-enhanced CT in PET/CT for the whole body in 12 subjects with different malignant disorders.[116] The study concluded that, despite the differences in AC, both methods correlated well in PET-positive lesions. However, the use of the Dixon sequence alone was not deemed to provide adequate anatomic information because of its low resolution, and the use of other MR sequences was encouraged.[116] In Hitz and colleagues,[117] the Dixon-based method was compared with CT-AC in 30 subjects with suspected dementia. Differences were observed in the PET/MR images compared with the PET/CT, but such differences "may only in part be explained by inconsistencies in the attenuation-correction procedures."[117]

The 3-class segmentation implemented on the Philips system was also clinically evaluated for head-and-neck cancers in 32 subjects with equivalent performance to PET/CT as reported in Varoquaux and colleagues.[118] In lymph node cancer it also showed "a strong parallel to PET/CT in terms of SUVmax, interobserver agreement and diagnostic performance."[119]

Finally, the use of PET/MR imaging with the UTE-based method was compared with PET/CT in 16 subjects with various neurologic indications. The study concluded that the "PET quantitation accuracy using the MR imaging based UTE sequences for AC in simultaneous brain PET/MR imaging is reliable in a clinical setting, being similar to that obtained using PET/CT."[71]

SUMMARY AND FUTURE OF ATTENUATION CORRECTION FOR PET/MR IMAGING

There has been an explosion of methods developed to overcome the challenging task of AC in PET/MR imaging scanners. Comparative studies very strongly suggest that bone attenuation needs to be accounted for not only for accurate quantification but also to avoid potential clinical misinterpretation. It seems that combined methods might provide more accurate and robust results as the synergistic combination of their strengths can be used to overcome their individual limitations.

Regarding artifacts (implants, truncation, and so forth), it is quite clear that more robust methods are required to reduce their effect on the final PET images. New MR sequences, such as ZT, MAVRIC, HUGE, and others, could potentially offer innovative solutions to overcome such problems and improve the MR-AC solutions.

Moving forward, MR-AC methods will need to be developed for more robust estimation of whole-body attenuation maps, particularly in the lungs.

REFERENCES

1. Keereman V, Mollet P, Berker Y, et al. Challenges and current methods for attenuation correction in PET/MR. MAGMA 2013;26:81–98.
2. Bezrukov I, Mantlik F, Schmidt H, et al. MR-based PET attenuation correction for PET/MR imaging. Semin Nucl Med 2013;43:45–59.
3. Huang SC, Hoffman EJ, Phelps ME, et al. Quantitation in positron emission computed tomography: 2. Effects of inaccurate attenuation correction. J Comput Assist Tomogr 1979;3:804–14.
4. Bergstrom M, Litton J, Eriksson L, et al. Determination of object contour from projections for attenuation correction in cranial positron emission tomography. J Comput Assist Tomogr 1982;6:365–72.
5. Weinzapfel BT, Hutchins GD. Automated PET attenuation correction model for functional brain imaging. J Nucl Med 2001;42:483–91.

time-of-flight PET. IEEE Trans Med Imaging 2012; 31:2224–33.

61. Defrise M, Rezaei A, Nuyts J. Time-of-flight PET data determine the attenuation sinogram up to a constant. Phys Med Biol 2012;57:885–99.

62. Mehranian A, Zaidi H. Joint estimation of activity and attenuation in whole-body TOF PET/MRI using constrained gaussian mixture models. IEEE Trans Med Imaging 2015;34(9):1808–21.

63. Mehranian A, Zaidi H. Clinical assessment of emission- and segmentation-based MR-guided attenuation correction in whole-body time-of-flight PET/MR imaging. J Nucl Med 2015;56:877–83.

64. Mollet P, Keereman V, Clementel E, et al. Simultaneous MR-compatible emission and transmission imaging for PET using time-of-flight information. IEEE Trans Med Imaging 2012;31:1734–42.

65. Mollet P, Keereman V, Bini J, et al. Improvement of attenuation correction in time-of-flight PET/MR imaging with a positron-emitting source. J Nucl Med 2014;55:329–36.

66. Bowen SL, Catana C. Transmission imaging for a simultaneous PET-MR system. IEEE Nucl. Sci. Symp. Conf. Seattle, WA, November 8–15, 2014.

67. Rothfuss H, Panin V, Moor A, et al. LSO background radiation as a transmission source using time of flight. Phys Med Biol 2014;59:5483–500.

68. Ouyang J, Chun SY, Petibon Y, et al. Bias atlases for segmentation-based PET attenuation correction using PET-CT and MR. IEEE Trans Nucl Sci 2013; 60:3373–82.

69. Izquierdo-Garcia D, Sawiak SJ, Knesaurek K, et al. Comparison of MR-based attenuation correction and CT-based attenuation correction of whole-body PET/MR imaging. Eur J Nucl Med Mol Imaging 2014;41:1574–84.

70. Marshall HR, Prato FS, Deans L, et al. Variable lung density consideration in attenuation correction of whole-body PET/MRI. J Nucl Med 2012;53:977–84.

71. Jena A, Taneja S, Goel R, et al. Reliability of semi-quantitative (1)(8)F-FDG PET parameters derived from simultaneous brain PET/MRI: a feasibility study. Eur J Radiol 2014;83:1269–74.

72. Yoon SH, Goo JM, Lee SM, et al. Positron emission tomography/magnetic resonance imaging evaluation of lung cancer: current status and future prospects. J Thorac Imaging 2014;29:4–16.

73. Catana C. Motion correction options in PET/MRI. Semin Nucl Med 2015;45:212–23.

74. Delso G, Martinez-Moller A, Bundschuh RA, et al. The effect of limited MR field of view in MR/PET attenuation correction. Med Phys 2010; 37:2804–12.

75. Schramm G, Langner J, Hofheinz F, et al. Influence and compensation of truncation artifacts in MR-based attenuation correction in PET/MR. IEEE Trans Med Imaging 2013;32:2056–63.

76. Nuyts J, Bal G, Kehren F, et al. Completion of a truncated attenuation image from the attenuated PET emission data. IEEE Trans Med Imaging 2013;32:237–46.

77. Blumhagen JO, Ladebeck R, Fenchel M, et al. MR-based field-of-view extension in MR/PET: B0 homogenization using gradient enhancement (HUGE). Magn Reson Med 2013;70:1047–57.

78. Blumhagen JO, Braun H, Ladebeck R, et al. Field of view extension and truncation correction for MR-based human attenuation correction in simultaneous MR/PET imaging. Med Phys 2014;41: 022303.

79. New PF, Rosen BR, Brady TJ, et al. Potential hazards and artifacts of ferromagnetic and nonferromagnetic surgical and dental materials and devices in nuclear magnetic resonance imaging. Radiology 1983;147:139–48.

80. Kinahan PE, Hasegawa BH, Beyer T. X-ray-based attenuation correction for positron emission tomography/computed tomography scanners. Semin Nucl Med 2003;33:166–79.

81. Ladefoged CN, Andersen FL, Keller SH, et al. PET/MR imaging of the pelvis in the presence of endoprostheses: reducing image artifacts and increasing accuracy through inpainting. Eur J Nucl Med Mol Imaging 2013;40:594–601.

82. Bezrukov I, Schmidt H, Mantlik F, et al. MR-based attenuation correction methods for improved PET quantification in lesions within bone and susceptibility artifact regions. J Nucl Med 2013;54:1768–74.

83. Burger IA, Wurnig MC, Becker AS, et al. Hybrid PET/MR imaging: an algorithm to reduce metal artifacts from dental implants in Dixon-based attenuation map generation using a multiacquisition variable-resonance image combination sequence. J Nucl Med 2015;56:93–7.

84. Lois C, Bezrukov I, Schmidt H, et al. Effect of MR contrast agents on quantitative accuracy of PET in combined whole-body PET/MR imaging. Eur J Nucl Med Mol Imaging 2012;39:1756–66.

85. Conti M. Why is TOF PET reconstruction a more robust method in the presence of inconsistent data? Phys Med Biol 2011;56:155–68.

86. Davison H, ter Voert EE, de Galiza Barbosa F, et al. Incorporation of time-of-flight information reduces metal artifacts in simultaneous positron emission tomography/magnetic resonance imaging: a simulation study. Invest Radiol 2015;50:423–9.

87. Mehranian A, Zaidi H. Impact of time-of-flight PET on quantification errors in MR imaging-based attenuation correction. J Nucl Med 2015;56:635–41.

88. Boellaard R, Hofman MB, Hoekstra OS, et al. Accurate PET/MR quantification using time of flight MLAA image reconstruction. Mol Imaging Biol 2014;16:469–77.

89. Delso G, Martinez-Moller A, Bundschuh RA, et al. Evaluation of the attenuation properties of MR equipment for its use in a whole-body PET/MR scanner. Phys Med Biol 2010;55:4361–74.

90. Tellmann L, Quick HH, Bockisch A, et al. The effect of MR surface coils on PET quantification in whole-body PET/MR: results from a pseudo-PET/MR phantom study. Med Phys 2011;38:2795–805.

91. MacDonald LR, Kohlmyer S, Liu C, et al. Effects of MR surface coils on PET quantification. Med Phys 2011;38:2948–56.

92. Wollenweber SD, Delso G, Deller T, et al. Characterization of the impact to PET quantification and image quality of an anterior array surface coil for PET/MR imaging. MAGMA 2014;27:149–59.

93. Paulus DH, Braun H, Aklan B, et al. Simultaneous PET/MR imaging: MR-based attenuation correction of local radiofrequency surface coils. Med Phys 2012;39:4306–15.

94. Paulus DH, Tellmann L, Quick HH. Towards improved hardware component attenuation correction in PET/MR hybrid imaging. Phys Med Biol 2013;58:8021–40.

95. Kartmann R, Paulus DH, Braun H, et al. Integrated PET/MR imaging: automatic attenuation correction of flexible RF coils. Med Phys 2013;40:082301.

96. Mantlik F, Hofmann M, Werner MK, et al. The effect of patient positioning aids on PET quantification in PET/MR imaging. Eur J Nucl Med Mol Imaging 2011;38:920–9.

97. Ferguson A, McConathy J, Su Y, et al. Attenuation effects of MR headphones during brain PET/MR studies. J Nucl Med Technol 2014;42:93–100.

98. Schleyer PJ, Schaeffter T, Marsden PK. The effect of inaccurate bone attenuation coefficient and segmentation on reconstructed PET images. Nucl Med Commun 2010;31:708–16.

99. Samarin A, Burger C, Wollenweber SD, et al. PET/MR imaging of bone lesions–implications for PET quantification from imperfect attenuation correction. Eur J Nucl Med Mol Imaging 2012;39: 1154–60.

100. Kim JH, Lee JS, Song IC, et al. Comparison of segmentation-based attenuation correction methods for PET/MRI: evaluation of bone and liver standardized uptake value with oncologic PET/CT data. J Nucl Med 2012;53:1878–82.

101. Akbarzadeh A, Ay MR, Ahmadian A, et al. MRI-guided attenuation correction in whole-body PET/MR: assessment of the effect of bone attenuation. Ann Nucl Med 2013;27:152–62.

102. Schramm G, Langner J, Hofheinz F, et al. Quantitative accuracy of attenuation correction in the Philips Ingenuity TF whole-body PET/MR system: a direct comparison with transmission-based attenuation correction. MAGMA 2013;26:115–26.

103. Partovi S, Kohan A, Gaeta C, et al. Image quality assessment of automatic three-segment MR attenuation correction vs. CT attenuation correction. Am J Nucl Med Mol Imaging 2013;3:291–9.

104. Bini J, Izquierdo-Garcia D, Mateo J, et al. Preclinical evaluation of MR attenuation correction versus CT attenuation correction on a sequential whole-body MR/PET scanner. Invest Radiol 2013;48: 313–22.

105. Andersen FL, Ladefoged CN, Beyer T, et al. Combined PET/MR imaging in neurology: MR-based attenuation correction implies a strong spatial bias when ignoring bone. Neuroimage 2014;84: 206–16.

106. Aznar MC, Sersar R, Saabye J, et al. Whole-body PET/MRI: the effect of bone attenuation during MR-based attenuation correction in oncology imaging. Eur J Radiol 2014;83:1177 83.

107. Brendle C, Schmidt H, Oergel A, et al. Segmentation-based attenuation correction in positron emission tomography/magnetic resonance: erroneous tissue identification and its impact on positron emission tomography interpretation. Invest Radiol 2015;50:339–46.

108. Dickson JC, O'Meara C, Barnes A. A comparison of CT- and MR-based attenuation correction in neurological PET. Eur J Nucl Med Mol Imaging 2014;41:1176–89.

109. Delso G, Carl M, Wiesinger F, et al. Anatomic evaluation of 3-dimensional ultrashort-echo-time bone maps for PET/MR attenuation correction. J Nucl Med 2014;55:780–5.

110. Arabi H, Rager O, Alem A, et al. Clinical assessment of MR-guided 3-class and 4-class attenuation correction in PET/MR. Mol Imaging Biol 2015;17: 264–76.

111. Keller SH, Holm S, Hansen AE, et al. Image artifacts from MR-based attenuation correction in clinical, whole-body PET/MRI. MAGMA 2013;26: 173–81.

112. Eiber M, Martinez-Moller A, Souvatzoglou M, et al. Value of a Dixon-based MR/PET attenuation correction sequence for the localization and evaluation of PET-positive lesions. Eur J Nucl Med Mol Imaging 2011;38:1691–701.

113. Drzezga A, Souvatzoglou M, Eiber M, et al. First clinical experience with integrated whole-body PET/MR: comparison to PET/CT in patients with oncologic diagnoses. J Nucl Med 2012; 53:845–55.

114. Fraum TJ, Fowler KJ, McConathy J, et al. PET/MRI for the body imager: abdominal and pelvic oncologic applications. Abdom Imaging 2015;40(6): 1387–404.

115. Schafer JF, Gatidis S, Schmidt H, et al. Simultaneous whole-body PET/MR imaging in comparison

to PET/CT in pediatric oncology: initial results. Radiology 2014;273:220–31.

116. Jeong JH, Cho IH, Kong EJ, et al. Evaluation of Dixon sequence on hybrid PET/MR compared with contrast-enhanced PET/CT for PET-positive lesions. Nucl Med Mol Imaging 2014; 48:26–32.

117. Hitz S, Habekost C, Furst S, et al. Systematic comparison of the performance of integrated whole-body PET/MR imaging to conventional PET/CT for 18F-FDG brain imaging in patients examined for suspected dementia. J Nucl Med 2014;55: 923–31.

118. Varoquaux A, Rager O, Poncet A, et al. Detection and quantification of focal uptake in head and neck tumours: (18)F-FDG PET/MR versus PET/CT. Eur J Nucl Med Mol Imaging 2014;41:462–75.

119. Kohan AA, Kolthammer JA, Vercher-Conejero JL, et al. N staging of lung cancer patients with PET/MRI using a three-segment model attenuation correction algorithm: initial experience. Eur Radiol 2013;23:3161–9.

Attenuation Correction for Magnetic Resonance Coils in Combined PET/MR Imaging: A Review

Mootaz Eldib, MS[a,b], Jason Bini, PhD[c], David D. Faul, PhD[d],
Niels Oesingmann, PhD[d], Charalampos Tsoumpas, PhD[a,e],
Zahi A. Fayad, PhD[a,f,g],*

KEYWORDS

- PET/MR imaging • Attenuation correction • MR imaging surface coils • PET/MR reconstruction
- Scatter correction • Image analysis

KEY POINTS

- MR imaging coils and imaging hardware could induce large quantitative errors and image artifacts; attenuation correction is needed.
- Computed tomography–based and transmission-based attenuation maps might be feasible for small coils, but not large ones.
- Attenuation correction for flexible coils that change position and shape between or during imaging sessions is still challenging.
- Degree of scattered events due to magnetic resonance coils and possible corrections has not yet been studied.
- Clinical evaluation of the attenuation of coils is challenging and requires more research and development.

INTRODUCTION

PET is a functional imaging technique that displays the bio-distribution of externally administered radioactive tracers to the body. The measurement of tracer concentrations down to picomolar concentrations is a unique advantage of PET.[1] However, several physical effects, such as attenuation, scatter, random coincidences, and detector efficiency normalization, must be accounted for in order to achieve an accurate quantification.[1,2]

Dr D.D. Faul and Dr N. Oesingmann are employed by Siemens Healthcare. Dr M. Eldib, Dr J. Bini, Dr C. Tsoumpas, and Dr Z.A. Fayad have nothing to disclose.
This work is supported in part by a grant from the National Institutes of Health, National Heart Lung and Blood Institute (NIH/NHLBI R01 HL071021) (Z.A. Fayad).
a Translational and Molecular Imaging Institute, Icahn School of Medicine at Mount Sinai, One Gustave L. Levy Place, New York, NY 10029, USA; b Department of Biomedical Engineering, The City College of New York, 160 Convent Avenue, New York, NY 10031, USA; c Department of Diagnostic Radiology, PET Center, Yale School of Medicine, Yale University, 801 Howard Avenue, New Haven, CT 06520, USA; d Siemens Healthcare, 527 Madison Avenue, New York, NY 10022, USA; e Division of Biomedical Imaging, Faculty of Medicine and Health, University of Leeds, 8.001a Worsley Building, Clarendon Way, Leeds LS2 9JT, UK; f Department of Radiology, Icahn School of Medicine at Mount Sinai, One Gustave L. Levy Place, New York, NY 10029, USA; g Department of Cardiology, Zena and Michael A. Weiner Cardiovascular Institute, Marie-Josée and Henry R. Kravis Cardiovascular Health Center, Icahn School of Medicine at Mount Sinai, One Gustave L. Levy Place, New York, NY 10029, USA
* Corresponding author. Translational and Molecular Imaging Institute, Icahn School of Medicine at Mount Sinai, One Gustave L. Levy Place, PO Box 1234, New York, NY 10029.
E-mail address: zahi.fayad@mssm.edu

PET Clin 11 (2016) 151–160
http://dx.doi.org/10.1016/j.cpet.2015.10.004
1556-8598/16/$ – see front matter © 2016 Elsevier Inc. All rights reserved.

Attenuation of PET photons by all objects in the field of view (FOV) is one of the major challenges of PET imaging, leading to the underestimation of tracer uptake and to image artifacts.[3] In all PET systems (ie, stand-alone, PET/computed tomography [CT], or PET/magnetic resonance [MR]), attenuation correction (AC) must be applied for the patient body, patient positioning aids (ie, cushions and pillows), as well as the patient table. PET/MR systems are unique because imaging coils such as head and neck, knee, cardiac, or carotid coils are used to detect the MR signal, as shown in **Fig. 1**.

To visualize the effect of attenuation on quantification, **Fig. 2**A shows an example of a fully corrected PET image for attenuation of both the patient and the MR hardware, including the patient table and the head and neck coil. If the attenuation for MR imaging hardware is not accounted for as in **Fig. 2**B, the measured uptake is considerably reduced. If the attenuation of the patient is not accounted for (**Fig. 2**C), an even larger error is observed. As a result, AC for all objects must be applied in order to quantify the tracer uptake accurately.

Hybrid PET scanners mainly exist as systems combined with either a CT or an MR scanner. In combined PET/CT systems, AC is performed using the CT data that is sequentially acquired during the same examination. In the case of PET/MR, the MR signal is unrelated to attenuation or electron density and thus cannot be directly used for AC. As a result, different AC strategies were needed depending on whether one is correcting for the attenuation of the patient or the MR hardware (ie, coils and patient table).[4–8] Several review articles have focused on AC methods for patients.[9–11] In this review article, currently published work on AC for MR coils and hardware are summarized.

Also limitations and opportunities to further develop methods and applications are discussed.

PET/MAGNETIC RESONANCE COILS

MR surface coils are electronic equipment that vary in size and shape depending on their application. They are made of a mix of materials including plastic and rubber, but most relevant are conducting materials for wiring and electronic circuitry. The attenuation of gamma rays is directly related to the electron density distribution of the material. Hence, it might be feasible to optimize the design of the MR coils with respect to lower attenuation properties and, when possible, with materials that do not affect the PET signal significantly. In a simulation study that aimed to recommend optimized configurations, it was found that plastics such as polytetrafluoroethylene are less suitable for coils than polyethylene for example.[12] It was also concluded that dense materials such as capacitors have a significant impact on attenuation and should be moved away from the patient. The findings of this simulation study were applied recently for a design of a PET/MR optimized head and neck coil.[13] The coil used thin plastic housing and thin copper wires and attempted to move the electronics as far away from the PET FOV as possible. The attenuation properties of the coil were compared with the standard head and neck coil. The optimized design of the coil resulted in significantly lower attenuation with a remaining 20% error in quantification.[13] Hence, even for optimized coil designs with least attenuation effects, the AC must not be omitted currently.

Additional studies were performed with optimized PET/MR coils such as the body matrix coil.[14] The

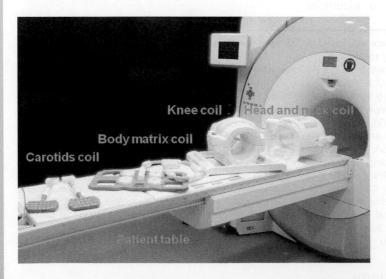

Fig. 1. Image of a biograph mMR along with several receiver coils.

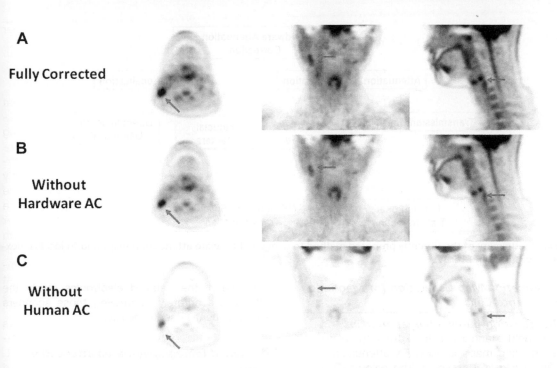

Fig. 2. Sample PET images with arrows pointing to a lesion in the neck. (*A*) Fully corrected PET image. (*B*) PET image reconstructed without account for the MR hardware, including the patient table and the head and neck coil. (*C*) PET image reconstructed without human AC.

use of the coil resulted in errors that reached 20% in areas near highly attenuating parts of the coil, which come in close proximity to the patient. The authors concluded that AC is required for the optimized body matrix coil.[15]

Taken together, although it is relevant to optimize the design of PET/MR coils with respect to attenuation, the design of completely PET-transparent coils is not yet possible and AC must be applied if they are to be used for quantitative PET examinations on the hybrid PET/MR scanner.[13,16]

ATTENUATION CORRECTION FOR MR IMAGING COILS

Although several MR-based methods have been proposed to correct for body tissue attenuation in combined PET/MR imaging, AC for MR coils, particularly flexible MR coils, remains an active area for research and development.[14,15,17–23] For rigid coils, such as the head and the spine matrix coils, the attenuation map can be generated, memorized, and used in the PET reconstruction whenever the specific portion of coils is within the FOV of the scan,[23] made possible because such coils retain their position in the PET FOV for all scans, allowing for the use a fixed template attenuation map for AC. Currently available commercial PET/MR

scanners use either transmission-based (TX) or CT-based attenuation maps for rigid MR hardware, which is discussed in the next section.[23,24] Flexible coils, on the other hand, change their shape and position from one imaging session to the next in adaptation to the size of the patient. In addition, the coils may move during the acquisition primarily because of physiologic or involuntary movements of the patient,[25] which makes the use of a fixed template attenuation map currently not feasible or impractical. Examples of flexible MR coils include cardiac coils, carotid coils, and the body matrix coil. By design, flexible MR coils are purposely invisible in conventional PET and MR imaging, which makes accurate localization of such coils in the PET FOV a challenging task. As a result of these challenges, AC for flexible coils is currently not implemented in commercially available PET/MR scanners despite the fact that significant attenuation of PET emission data can occur.[14,15,17,18,26,27]

Therefore, AC for MR hardware is a 2-step problem where (1) an attenuation map must be generated, and (2) for flexible coils, the coil must be localized in the PET FOV and the attenuation map must be aligned with the emission data. A summary of the proposed methods is shown in **Fig. 3**. Details of each method are further discussed in the later sections.

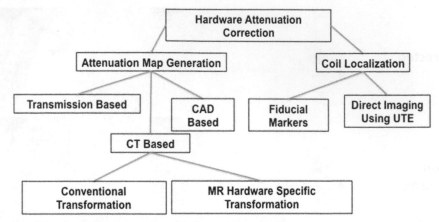

Fig. 3. Summary of the currently proposed method to generate hardware attenuation maps and to localize flexible coils in the PET FOV.

Attenuation Map Generation for Magnetic Resonance Coils

Transmission-based attenuation maps

The gold standard method for generating PET attenuation maps is using TX attenuation maps with a 511-keV source.[28] The calculation of TX attenuation maps is obtained by performing a blank scan without the object in the FOV and a transmission scan with the subject in the FOV. The attenuation correction factors are the ratio between the transmission scan and the blank scan, which is converted back to image space.[28] Typically, transmission attenuation maps are generated using a rotating 511-keV source that has a long half-life such as germanium-68. TX attenuation maps for MR coils and hardware are the standard AC method for the Philips Ingenuity TF PET/MR system (Philips Ingenuity, Cleveland, OH, USA).[23] The attenuation maps are stored as templates and are used for reconstruction whenever a specific part of the coil is within the PET FOV. The authors evaluated the accuracy of this TX attenuation map for the head and found that ignoring the attenuation of the coil resulted in about a 15% error.[23]

In order to provide TX AC for all objects in the FOV of a sequential PET/MR scanner, a transmission ring was mounted inside the bore of the PET scanner and allowed accurate AC for both the MR coils and the patient.[29] This method eliminates the need to pregenerate and store templates of the attenuation maps on the scanner and would also provide AC for flexible coils. A drawback is that it requires time-of-flight information during PET acquisitions.

Although TX-AC is the gold standard, it suffers from some limitations. PET scanners with a transmission source are generally older systems that are equipped with large-sized detector elements. The resultant spatial resolution of the attenuation map is not high enough in order to capture the structure of the detailed electronics inside the MR coils accurately. Moreover, those scanners are infrequently used clinically.

Computed tomography-based attenuation maps

The advent of combined PET/CT prompted the development of CT-based AC (CTAC).[30–32] CT imaging is a transmission imaging technique with a radiograph beam that contains photons of various energies from 10 to 100 KeV.[31] The Hounsfield units in CT images must be scaled to match the energy of the PET photons (511 KeV) in order to obtain a suitable AC. This scaling was experimentally measured and is approximated with a linear or a bilinear transformation.[32] A sample transmission and CT-based attenuation map of the patient beds are shown in **Fig. 4**.

CTAC has been used for AC of MR coils and hardware in hybrid PET/MR scanners[13,14,17,20,33,34] and constitutes the most common and most tested method for producing hardware attenuation maps. This approach for AC is currently used on the Siemens Biograph mMR.[14,24]

Several studies have evaluated the feasibility of CTAC and have reported contradicting results. For example, Aklan and colleagues[35] reported that CTAC was accurate for a breast coil. Moreover, Paulus and colleagues[14] reported successful AC for the body matrix coil.[18] Very recently, Dregely and colleagues[16] reported accurate AC using a CT-based map for a new PET/MR optimized breast coil. On the other hand, MacDonald and colleagues[20] reported that CTAC resulted in artifacts and overcorrection in the reconstructed PET image using a head and neck coil. Furthermore, Delso and colleagues[33] reported localized errors when attempting to correct for a different head and neck coil using a CT-based attenuation map.

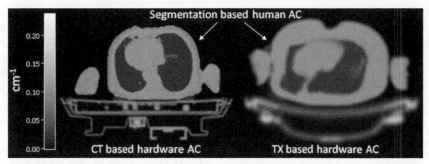

Fig. 4. Sample transmission- and CT-based attenuation maps of the patient table.

Studies with CTAC concluded that most of the errors emanated from metal and beam hardening artifacts in the attenuation maps.[33] To address these errors, some studies applied an empirically defined threshold on the CT-based attenuation maps and showed the possible elimination of errors caused by metal and beam-hardening artifacts.[17,35] Although these methods could help, **Fig. 5** shows

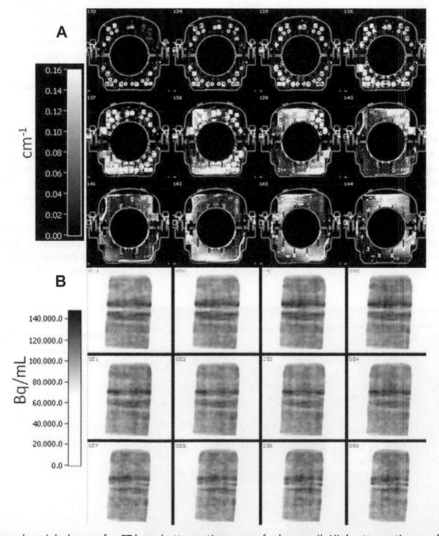

Fig. 5. (A) Sample axial planes of a CT-based attenuation map of a knee coil. High-attenuation coefficients and metal artifacts can be seen. (B) Sample coronal planes from the PET image volume reconstructed with the attenuation map shown in the (A). AC-induced image artifacts and quantitative error as can be seen in the image.

an example CT-based attenuation map of a knee coil that contains a substantial amount of metal leading to several image artifacts. Consequently, the reconstructed PET image contains artifacts as shown in the bottom panel in **Fig. 5**.

Another concern in using CTAC is that the bilinear transformation from Hounsfield units to PET attenuation coefficients was developed for biological tissues and not for plastics and metals that are used in MR coils and hardware.[32] A study by Paulus and colleagues[19] attempted to develop a new MR-hardware specific transformation from Hounsfield units to PET attenuation coefficients and reported minor improvement in the quantification.

Taken together, CTAC for MR coils seems to be better suited for smaller coils that do not contain much metal or are made from dense materials.[17,18] For bulky constructions, however, CT-based attenuation maps may contain significant artifacts capable of inducing quantitative errors in the PET image. Those coil designs benefit most from an optimization of their construction.

Computer-aided design–based attenuation maps

MR coils are generally constructed of a few homogenous materials that have the same attenuation properties. In the design process of such coils, computer-aided design (CAD) drawings are generally used. These CAD drawings of each component of the coil could be described by small volume elements with the appropriate attenuation coefficients assigned.[34] The advantage of this approach is that the attenuation maps are of high resolution and free from artifacts. The limitation, however, is that this is only feasible for coils with a relatively small number of components.

Nevertheless, this AC approach was tested for the patient table of the Biograph mMR, but did not provide improved AC compared with the system standard CT-based attenuation map. A sample CAD-based attenuation map as compared with a CT-based attenuation map of the mMR patient table is shown in **Fig. 6**.

Localization of the Coils in the PET Field of View

Rigid coils, such as the head and neck coil for example, retain their position from one scan to another, and thus, the same attenuation map could be used during every scan. Flexible coils, on the other hand, change shape and position between and during each scan. Moreover, these coils are invisible in conventional PET/MR imaging and new approaches must be used to localize them accurately. Several groups have investigated the accuracy of AC related to the error in the localization of the coils. It was concluded that although the needed accuracy depends on the coil used, an error of about 3 to 4 mm is acceptable.[17,19,33] In the next sections, methods to localize coils in the PET FOV are summarized.

Markers-based localization

The simplest approach to localize MR coils in the FOV is by placing MR visible fiducial markers on their surface.[14,17,18,36] These markers must also be visible in the attenuation map, allowing for the registration of a template attenuation map, as shown in **Fig. 7**.

For flexible coils, the use of nonrigid registration algorithms has been proposed to register the attenuation map to the position of the markers in a particular examination.[17,18] Using this AC

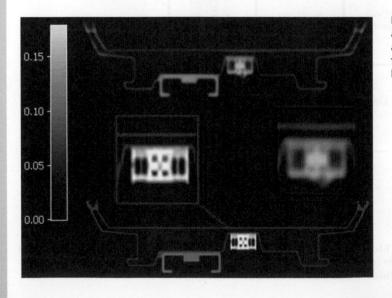

Fig. 6. (*top*) Sample CT-based attenuation map. (*bottom*) CAD-based attenuation map of the mMR patient table. (*insets*) Some artifacts in the CT-based attenuation map.

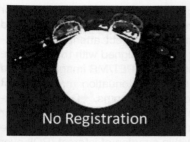
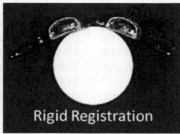
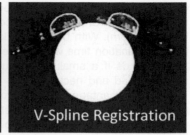

Fig. 7. Overlap between the reference position shown in the fire color map and the attenuation map to be registered by fiducial markers in the rainbow color map. (*left*) Overlap before registration. (*middle*) Overlap after rigid registration. (*right*) Overall after rigid and nonrigid registration using the volume spline algorithm (V-spline).

approach, the use of template-based AC for flexible coils could be used in routine clinical scans if the registration procedure is automated. A few studies have evaluated the feasibility of such algorithms and have found acceptable alignments within about 3 mm using a CT-based attenuation map, as shown in **Fig. 7**. The advantage of these approaches is that they are simple to implement in the clinical setting. Fiducial markers, however, may interfere with all MR images that are generated with the coil, and the physician must be aware of their presence before reading the data. Furthermore, the markers must remain fixed to the coil, which is currently inconvenient for routine use.[36] Moreover, fiducial marker-based registration uses a small set of scattered points in corresponding MR images, and thus, interpolation between those points must be used to estimate the position of the coil in the FOV. It was shown that significant misregistration could occur depending on the type of interpolation used, leading

to erroneous AC and quantitative errors in the reconstructed PET image.[17] Taken together, localization of flexible coils by fiducial markers is a feasible, although not ideal, technique.

Ultrashort echo time–based localization

Due to the limitations of fiducial marker-based localization of flexible coils, direct imaging of some of the components of the coil using an ultrashort echo time sequence (UTE) has been proposed as a method to localize coils in the PET FOV.[4,14,26] The UTE sequence is capable of visualizing solid materials such as polymeric plastic and bone.[37,38] It was shown that AC could be performed by automated nonrigid registration of a template attenuation map to the UTE image, making this method clinically feasible.[26] This method requires, however, that the coil be constructed specifically from materials that are known to exhibit a signal in the UTE image, as shown in **Fig. 8**, *top*. Using nonrigid registration, a

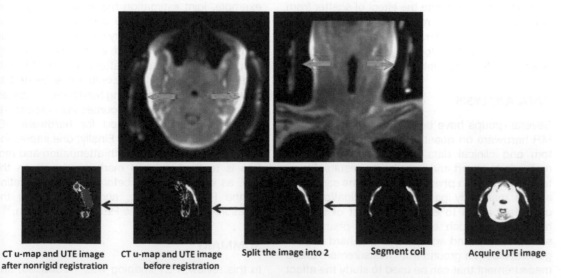

CT u-map and UTE image after nonrigid registration   CT u-map and UTE image before registration   Split the image into 2   Segment coil   Acquire UTE image

Fig. 8. (*top*) Coils could be imaged using the UTE sequence to localize the coil in the PET FOV as pointed out by the arrows. (*bottom*) Registration procedure to align a CT-based attenuation map.

CT-based attenuation map can be registered to the UTE image of the coil for accurate AC (see **Fig. 8**; *bottom*). With UTE-based localization, the total examination time will be extended by about 100 seconds if a small FOV is used, as in the case of head and neck imaging, for example.[26] The major advantage of this approach is that the registration could be more robust as compared with a fiducial markers–based registration due to the potential high degree of correlation between direct imaging of the entire coil and the attenuation map.

SCATTER CORRECTION FOR MAGNETIC RESONANCE COILS

An important physical effect that must be corrected for is the scattering of true coincidence events from interaction with the patient or the imaging hardware. In 3-dimensional PET, which is the current data acquisition approach, the scattered events must be subtracted to ensure accurate quantification of measured PET emission data.[39] Several algorithms have been developed to estimate the amount of scatter, such as the Gaussian fitting approaches or the model-based single-scatter simulation approach.[40,41] Scatter correction methods, however, do use the attenuation map of objects in the FOV to estimate the amount of scattered events. Consequently, the accuracy of the MR coils and imaging hardware attenuation map could play an important role in the scatter correction step. To the best of the authors' knowledge, no study has evaluated the effect of coil attenuation maps on the estimated scatter. The main reason for this is that it is difficult to experimentally isolate the effect of scatter from attenuation, and as a result, most studies merge the 2 effects together. The use of simulations could be a valuable tool to isolate the effect of scatter to study its contribution independently.

DATA ANALYSIS

Several groups have been studying the effect of MR hardware on quantification using both phantom and clinical data, which led to variety of methods to report and visualize the results. Phantom data, using a phantom of about the same size as the real body part under investigation, is a useful approach to isolate the effect of the MR hardware. In such experiments, a phantom is scanned with and without the MR hardware to generate both a ground truth measurement and a measurement that can be used to study the effect of the MR hardware as well as the feasibility of various data correction approaches. An important

aspect in using phantom measurements successfully is to insure that the attenuation map for the phantom contains the correct attenuation coefficients and that it is well aligned with the emission. This issue is relevant for PET/MR imagings where the system-generated attenuation maps are not designed to work for phantoms.[42] Data visualization in the phantom scans is often performed either by displaying a difference image or by plotting the mean activity within a region of interest (ROI) over all planes in the phantom, which provides a volumetric evaluation of the attenuation profile rather than just one plane. Instead, using a ROI about the same size of the anatomy of interest is suggested. Moreover, using uniform phantoms might be more desirable versus those that contain hot or cold regions so that the effect of attenuation is isolated from partial volume errors.

Another important aspect is to evaluate the effect of the MR hardware on quantification in clinical studies. Similar data collection is used as in the case of phantoms scans, where the subject is scanned with and without the MR hardware under investigation. A limitation to such method in human studies is that there might be a redistribution of the activity in between scans, and thus, the measurement differences could not be only due to the presence of the MR hardware. Because of this important limitation, interpretation of such data remains difficult.

FUTURE APPROACHES

Some AC methods have been proposed to correct for attenuation of the patient but could also extend to be used for MR coils and hardware. For example, joint estimation methods that estimate both the attenuation map and the PET image have been gaining popularity recently.[43,44] In addition, the use of scattered events was recently proposed to estimate the attenuation coefficients in PET/MR imaging and could be extended to include MR coils and imaging hardware.[45] Furthermore, placing low activity sources in or around the gantry could also be used for hardware AC, including flexible coils.[46,47] Finally, one interesting approach to correct for both attenuation and motion is to track fiducial markers placed on the coil, as was discussed before, over the duration of the PET acquisition, and incorporating the measured motion into the PET reconstruction.[48]

SUMMARY

In this review, PET imaging was introduced, and some of the problems of hardware AC for PET/MR were defined. These problems are currently not well addressed and require further research and development as well as clinical evaluation. The construction of PET transparent coils has proven insufficient, and AC is needed for an accurate quantification. TX-based AC appears to be well suited for AC for MR imaging hardware; however, clinical evaluation in humans has not been reported yet. The lack of availability of transmission scanners has made it difficult for researchers to test their feasibility. CT-based attenuation maps are easily generated, but they could contain artifacts and were shown to produce inconsistent results depending on the construction of the coil. It is possible, however, that the current lack of optimized acquisition, reconstruction, and thresholding parameters for CT-based maps could be the cause of the contradicting findings and must be further studied.

AC for flexible coils is still not accounted for in commercial PET/MR scanners, although they were shown to produce local errors up to 20%. Registration-based methods have been the most successful in this regard. Fiducial marker-based localization is not ideal clinically and may not produce accurate registration if the markers are placed sparsely or far away from critical components of the coil. Direct imaging of the hardware components using sequences like the UTE requires modification of some coils and increases scan time. With this in mind, progress is still needed in hardware AC to ensure the quantitative accuracy of PET/MR examinations.

ACKNOWLEDGMENTS

The authors thank Siemens Healthcare for its technical support.

REFERENCES

1. Wehrl HF, Sauter AW, Divine MR, et al. Combined PET/MR: a technology becomes mature. J Nucl Med 2015;56(2):165–8.
2. Fahey FH. Data acquisition in PET imaging. J Nucl Med Technol 2002;30(2):39–49.
3. Blodgett TM, Mehta AS, Mehta AS, et al. PET/CT artifacts. Clin Imaging 2011;35(1):49–63.
4. Mantlik F, Hofmann M, Werner MK, et al. The effect of patient positioning aids on PET quantification in PET/MR imaging. Eur J Nucl Med Mol Imaging 2011;38(5):920–9.
5. Bini J, Robson PM, Calcagno C, et al. Quantitative carotid PET/MR imaging: clinical evaluation of MR-attenuation correction versus CT-attenuation correction in (18)F-FDG PET/MR emission data and comparison to PET/CT. Am J Nucl Med Mol Imaging 2015;5(3):293–304.
6. Bini J, Eldib M, Robson PM, et al. Simultaneous carotid PET/MR: feasibility and improvement of magnetic resonance-based attenuation correction. Int J Cardiovasc Imaging 2015;11:1–11. [Epub ahead of print].
7. Aitken AP, Giese D, Tsoumpas C, et al. Improved UTE-based attenuation correction for cranial PET-MR using dynamic magnetic field monitoring. Med Phys 2014;41(1):012302.
8. Paulus DH, Thorwath D, Schmidt H, et al. Towards integration of PET/MR hybrid imaging into radiation therapy treatment planning. Med Phys 2014;41(7):072505.
9. Izquierdo-Garcia D, Catana C. Magnetic resonance imaging-guided attenuation correction of positron emission tomography data in PET/MRI. PET Clin, in press.
10. Wagenknecht G, Kaiser HJ, Mottaghy FM, et al. MRI for attenuation correction in PET: methods and challenges. MAGMA 2013;26(1):99–113.
11. Hofmann M, Pichler B, Scholkopf B, et al. Towards quantitative PET/MRI: a review of MR-based attenuation correction techniques. Eur J Nucl Med Mol Imaging 2009;36(Suppl 1):S93–104.
12. Herrick PDE, Ansorge RE, Hawkes RC, et al. Radiofrequency coil design for simultaneous PET/MR systems. Paper presented at Nuclear Science Symposium Conference Record (NSS/MIC), 2010 IEEE. Knoxville, TN, October 30, 2010–November 6, 2010.
13. Sander CY, Keil B, Chonde DB, et al. A 31-channel MR brain array coil compatible with positron emission tomography. Magn Reson Med 2015;73(6):2363–75.
14. Paulus DH, Braun H, Aklan B, et al. Simultaneous PET/MR imaging: MR-based attenuation correction of local radiofrequency surface coils. Med Phys 2012;39(7):4306–15.
15. Furst S, Souvatzoglou M, Martinez-Moller A, et al. Impact of flexible body surface coil and patient table on PET quantification and image quality in integrated PET/MR. Nuklearmedizin 2014;53(3):79–87.
16. Dregely I, Lanz T, Metz S, et al. A 16-channel MR coil for simultaneous PET/MR imaging in breast cancer. Eur Radiol 2015;25(4):1154–61.
17. Eldib M, Bini J, Calcagno C, et al. Attenuation correction for flexible magnetic resonance coils in combined magnetic resonance/positron emission tomography imaging. Invest Radiol 2014;49(2):63–9.
18. Kartmann R, Paulus DH, Braun H, et al. Integrated PET/MR imaging: automatic attenuation correction of flexible RF coils. Med Phys 2013;40(8):082301.
19. Paulus DH, Tellmann L, Quick HH. Towards improved hardware component attenuation correction in PET/MR hybrid imaging. Phys Med Biol 2013;58(22):8021–40.
20. MacDonald LR, Kohlmyer S, Liu C, et al. Effects of MR surface coils on PET quantification. Med Phys 2011;38(6):2948–56.

21. Wollenweber SD, Delso G, Deller T, et al. Characterization of the impact to PET quantification and image quality of an anterior array surface coil for PET/MR imaging. Magma 2013;27(2):149–59.

22. Tellmann L, Quick HH, Bockisch A, et al. The effect of MR surface coils on PET quantification in whole-body PET/MR: results from a pseudo-PET/MR phantom study. Med Phys 2011;38(5):2795–805.

23. Bin Z, Pal D, Zhiqiang H, et al. Attenuation correction for MR table and coils for a sequential PET/MR system. Paper presented at Nuclear Science Symposium Conference Record (NSS/MIC), 2009 IEEE. Orlando, FL, October 24, 2009–November 1, 2009.

24. Eldib M, Faul D, Pawlak J, et al. Verification of the MR components attenuation maps for an MR/PET scanner with simultaneous acquisition. J Nucl Med 2012;53(1_MeetingAbstracts):2331.

25. Kolbitsch C, Prieto C, Tsoumpas C, et al. 3D MR-acquisition scheme for nonrigid bulk motion correction in simultaneous PET-MR. Med Phys 2014;41(8):082304.

26. Eldib M, Bini J, Robson PM, et al. Markerless attenuation correction for carotid MRI surface receiver coils in combined PET/MR imaging. Phys Med Biol 2015;60(12):4705–17.

27. Ouyang J, Petibon Y, Huang C, et al. Quantitative simultaneous PET-MR imaging. J Med Imaging (Bellingham) 2014;9083:908325.

28. Bailey DL. Transmission scanning in emission tomography. Eur J Nucl Med 1998;25(7):774–87.

29. Mollet P, Keereman V, Bini J, et al. Improvement of attenuation correction in time-of-flight PET/MR imaging with a positron-emitting source. J Nucl Med 2014;55(2):329–36.

30. Kinahan PE, Hasegawa BH, Beyer T. X-ray-based attenuation correction for positron emission tomography/computed tomography scanners. Semin Nucl Med 2003;33(3):166–79.

31. Kinahan PE, Townsend DW, Beyer T, et al. Attenuation correction for a combined 3D PET/CT scanner. Med Phys 1998;25(10):2046–53.

32. Carney JP, Townsend DW, Rappoport V, et al. Method for transforming CT images for attenuation correction in PET/CT imaging. Med Phys 2006;33(4):976–83.

33. Delso G, Martinez-Moller A, Bundschuh RA, et al. Evaluation of the attenuation properties of MR equipment for its use in a whole-body PET/MR scanner. Phys Med Biol 2010;55(15):4361–74.

34. Eldib M, Faul D, Ladebeck R, et al. A method for estimating the attenuation correction for the MR hardware of an MR/PET scanner. J Nucl Med 2012;53(1_MeetingAbstracts):371.

35. Aklan B, Paulus DH, Wenkel E, et al. Toward simultaneous PET/MR breast imaging: systematic evaluation and integration of a radiofrequency breast coil. Med Phys 2013;40(2):024301.

36. Ferguson A, McConathy J, Su Y, et al. Attenuation effects of MR headphones during brain PET/MR studies. J Nucl Med Technol 2014;42(2):93–100.

37. Springer F, Martirosian P, Schwenzer NF, et al. Three-dimensional ultrashort echo time imaging of solid polymers on a 3-Tesla whole-body MRI scanner. Invest Radiol 2008;43(11):802–8.

38. Delso G, Carl M, Wiesinger F, et al. Anatomic evaluation of 3-dimensional ultrashort-echo-time bone maps for PET/MR attenuation correction. J Nucl Med 2014;55(5):780–5.

39. Ollinger JM. Model-based scatter correction for fully 3D PET. Phys Med Biol 1996;41(1):153–76.

40. Cherry SR, Huang SC. Effects of scatter on model parameter estimates in 3D PET studies of the human brain. IEEE Trans Nucl Sci 1995;42(4):1174–9.

41. Markiewicz PJ, Tamal M, Julyan PJ, et al. High accuracy multiple scatter modelling for 3D whole body PET. Phys Med Biol 2007;52(3):829–47.

42. Ziegler S, Braun H, Ritt P, et al. Systematic evaluation of phantom fluids for simultaneous PET/MR hybrid imaging. J Nucl Med 2013;54(8):1464–71.

43. Mehranian A, Zaidi H. Joint estimation of activity and attenuation in whole-body TOF PET/MRI using constrained Gaussian mixture models. IEEE Trans Med Imaging 2015;34(9):1808–21.

44. Mehranian A, Zaidi H. Emission-based estimation of lung attenuation coefficients for attenuation correction in time-of-flight PET/MR. Phys Med Biol 2015;60(12):4813–33.

45. Berker Y, Kiessling F, Schulz V. Scattered PET data for attenuation-map reconstruction in PET/MRI. Med Phys 2014;41(10):102502.

46. Watson C. Imaging the attenuation coefficients of positron beams in matter: positron attenuation tomography. EJNMMI Phys 2015;2(Suppl 1):A20.

47. Watson CC, Eriksson L, Kolb A. Physics and applications of positron beams in an integrated PET/MR. Phys Med Biol 2013;58(3):L1–12.

48. Huang C, Ackerman JL, Petibon Y, et al. Motion compensation for brain PET imaging using wireless MR active markers in simultaneous PET-MR: phantom and non-human primate studies. NeuroImage 2014;91:129–37.

MR Imaging–Guided Partial Volume Correction of PET Data in PET/MR Imaging

Kjell Erlandsson, PhD[a],*, John Dickson, PhD[b],
Simon Arridge, PhD[c], David Atkinson, PhD[d],
Sebastien Ourselin, PhD[e], Brian F. Hutton, PhD[a,f]

KEYWORDS

- Partial volume effects • Partial volume correction • PET/MR imaging • Quantification

KEY POINTS

- Partial volume correction (PVC) is important for accurate quantification in PET and for avoiding confounding factors related to changes in partial volume effects (PVEs) but is currently not routinely used in clinical practice.
- Coregistered anatomic information from MR imaging can be used for accurate PVC of PET data.
- Anatomically guided correction for PVEs can be performed as a postreconstruction procedure or during the image reconstruction process.
- The introduction of PET/MR imaging scanners could facilitate the use of PVC in routine clinical studies.

INTRODUCTION

Partial volume effects (PVEs) are caused by the limited spatial resolution of the PET system, which results in a blurry appearance of the reconstructed PET images and, as a consequence, a reduction in the observed maximum activity for small objects[1] (Box 1). Partial volume correction (PVC) is essential for accurate quantification in PET, especially in small objects. PVC can also be important in situations when the PVE changes over time or between subjects (Box 2).

PVEs can be regarded as 2 separate effects: spill-out of data from inside an image region and spill-in of data from outside into the region. The amount of spill-over between regions depends on the point-spread function (PSF) of the imaging system, which is often modeled as a 3-dimensional Gaussian function, characterized by its full-width at half-maximum (FWHM): the larger the FWHM, the larger the spillover. The blurring of the reconstructed PET distribution can be described by an integral transform, which, if the PSF is position invariant, is called convolution. In principle, it is

The authors have nothing to disclose.

The amyloid and fludeoxyglucose PET images shown were from a study supported by AVID Radiopharmaceuticals (a wholly owned subsidiary of Eli Lilly) and the National Brain Appeal, Frontotemporal Dementia Research Fund. This work was supported by the EPSRC (grant number EP/K005278/1), the EC under the FP7 INSERT project (grant number 305311), and the National Institute for Health Research University College London Hospitals Biomedical Research Center.

[a] Institute of Nuclear Medicine, University College London, UCLH, Euston Road (T-5), London NW1 2BU, UK; [b] Institute of Nuclear Medicine, University College London Hospital, UCLH, Euston Road (T-5), London NW1 2BU, UK; [c] Department of Computer Science, University College London, Gower Street, London WC1E 6BT, UK; [d] Centre for Medical Imaging, University College London, 250 Euston Road, London NW1 2PG, UK; [e] Centre for Medical Imaging Computing, University College London, Gower Street, London WC1E 6BT, UK; [f] The Centre for Medical Radiation Physics, University of Wollongong, Northfields Avenue, Wollongong NSW 2522, Australia
* Corresponding author. UCLH, Euston Road (T-5), London NW1 2BU, UK.
E-mail address: k.erlandsson@ucl.ac.uk

PET Clin 11 (2016) 161–177
http://dx.doi.org/10.1016/j.cpet.2015.09.002

Box 1
The PVE

Fig. 1 shows results from a simulated National Electrical Manufacturers Association-International Electrotechnical Commission (NEMA-IEC) phantom. The highest value in the largest spheres is correct in the noise-free case; but for the smaller spheres, the maximum value decreases as the diameter decreases. The true values in all the spheres can be restored by partial volume correction.

Fig. 2 shows the maximum (max) and mean values as a function of diameter. With noisy data, the max value gives overestimation for the larger spheres and underestimation for the smaller spheres, whereas the mean value gives underestimation for all spheres and is much less sensitive to noise.

---

possible to reduce the severity of the PVEs by performing an inverse filtering or deconvolution operation on the reconstructed image[2,3] or by using a resolution recovery technique during image reconstruction.[4,5] However, this type of method cannot provide a full correction because of the loss of high-frequency information from the measured PET data. In order to perform a more accurate correction for PVEs, it is necessary to introduce additional information, which can be obtained from high-resolution anatomic images, such as computed tomography (CT) or MR imaging. Several correction methods based on anatomic images have been developed in the past, although these are not in general being used routinely in

clinical practice. Various reviews of PVC methods have been published previously.[1,6,7]

In anatomically guided PVC methods, the anatomic image must, first of all, be coregistered with the PET image. Furthermore, most methods require that it be segmented into regions, which, for the purpose of the correction, can be assumed to contain a uniform distribution of activity. The result of the PVC is sensitive to errors in the coregistration and segmentation steps.[8–10] The image coregistration can be performed with a range of available software tools,[11–13] but it obviously becomes easier if the images have been acquired on a multimodality system, such as PET/CT or PET/MR imaging.[14,15] With a PET/CT scanner, the CT scan and the PET data acquisition are actually performed sequentially, so there is a possibility of patient motion between the two. On the other hand, a PET/MR imaging scanner technically allows for truly simultaneous acquisition of PET and MR imaging data. Although coregistration may still be needed, the adjustment needed should be minimal and any residual errors small. With regard to segmentation, MR imaging is in general preferable to CT, as it has better soft tissue contrast, which is especially important in brain studies. For these reasons, the recent introduction of PET/MR imaging scanners could greatly facilitate the use of PVC in routine clinical studies.

PARTIAL VOLUME CORRECTION METHODS

The correction for PVEs based on anatomic data can be considered to fall into 2 main

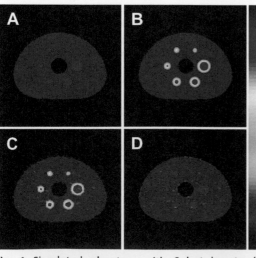

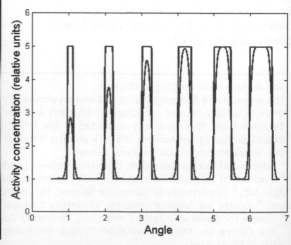

Fig. 1. Simulated phantom with 6 hot inserts. (*Left panel*) Original phantom (*A*), reconstructed image without noise (*B*) and with noise, before (*C*) and after partial volume correction with region-based voxelwise correction[16] (*D*). (*Right panel*) A circular profile through the center of the spheres in the original phantom (*blue line*) and in the reconstructed image without noise (*red line*).

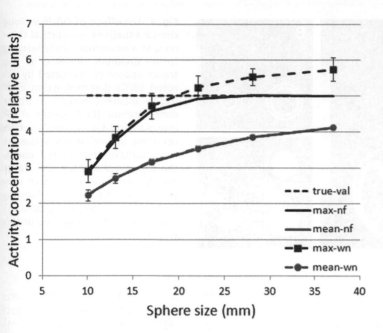

Fig. 2. Maximum (*blue lines*) and mean values (val) (*red lines*) in the spherical inserts as a function of sphere-size for noise-free data (nf; *solid lines*) and data with noise (wn; *dashed lines*).

approaches: postreconstruction methods and reconstruction-based methods. A brief historical overview of these methods is presented as well as a review of the findings for various clinical applications. Of the 2 main approaches, the postreconstruction methods appeared first. Initially the correction was applied to the mean value for one or more volumes of interest (VOIs), and later voxel-by-voxel methods were developed. The next step was to incorporate anatomic information directly into the image reconstruction algorithm. It has been shown that the reconstruction-based methods can be superior in terms of bias versus noise trade-off.[17] On the other hand, the postreconstruction methods have the advantage of being easier to implement and can be combined with the standard reconstruction software

provided with the system. The historical evolution of the different methods is shown in **Fig. 4**.

Postreconstruction Methods

In 1979, Hoffman and colleagues[18] proposed a method to correct the mean value in an image region or VOI, assuming a uniform distribution within the VOI and no background activity. The corrected value was obtained by dividing the uncorrected mean value by a precalculated recovery coefficient (RC), which depended on the shape and size of the VOI and the system PSF. This method corrected for spill-out but not for spill-in. From here, multiple PVC methods evolved in different directions. RC-based methods have often been used for PVC in oncology.[19]

Regional simultaneous estimation methods (A)

A series of method were developed, based on the principle of simultaneously estimating the mean values in 2 or more regions by first calculating the RCs for all regions and the crosstalk coefficients for all combinations of regions and then solving a system of linear equations. This approach corrected for both spill-in and spill-out. In 1983, Henze and colleagues[20] developed a PVC method for cardiac studies, with simultaneous estimation of the activity concentrations in the myocardial wall and the ventricular cavity of the left ventricle. Four recovery/crosstalk coefficients were determined, based on the geometry of the heart and the system PSF; the corrected mean values were obtained by solving a system

---

Box 2
Clinical PVEs

PVC can be important in situations when the PVEs change over time or between subjects and could be a confounding factor in the interpretation of the PET images.

In neurology studies of patients with Alzheimer disease, atrophy can lead to thinning of the cortical gray matter layer as compared with normal subjects (**Fig. 3**A). In cardiology studies, the thickness of the myocardial wall changes during the cardiac cycle, being thicker at end-systole as compared with end-diastole (**Fig. 3**B). In oncology studies, the size of a tumor can change after therapy (**Fig. 3**C).

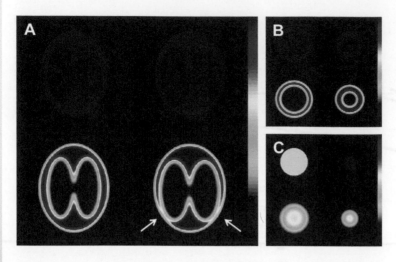

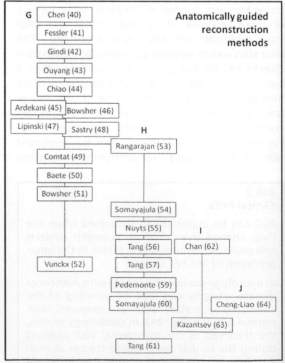

Fig. 3. The effects of PVE in various clinical situations. (*A*) Cortical thinning in a neurologic study leading to an apparent decrease in the tracer uptake (as indicated by *arrows*). (*B*) Cardiac contraction leading to apparent increase in tracer concentration. (*C*) A change in tumor size and tracer concentration resulting in unchanged apparent mean concentration. In each panel, the top row shows the true tracer distribution, and the bottom row shows the PVE-affected distributions. The left and right columns show anatomic changes occurring over time.

of 2 linear equations with 2 unknowns, assuming no background activity. In 1998, Rousset and colleagues[21] presented a similar method for neurology but with many more regions, covering the entire brain. A matrix of recovery/crosstalk coefficients was generated (the geometric transfer matrix [GTM]), and the corrected mean values of all regions were obtained by multiplying the inverse of this matrix with a column-vector containing the uncorrected mean values. This method is known as the GTM method. Labbé and colleagues[22] presented a similar method. Here the image was modeled as the sum of several components, each one corresponding to a single region convolved with the system PSF, multiplied by unknown coefficients. The investigators used

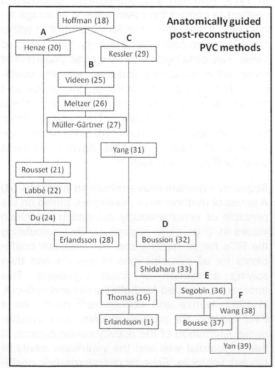

Fig. 4. The historical development of anatomically guided postreconstruction PVC methods (*left*) and reconstruction-based methods incorporating anatomic data (*right*). (The letters A–J refer to corresponding sections in the text.)

singular value decomposition to determine the values of the coefficients, which represent the corrected mean values for the different regions; but other mathematical techniques could be used. For example, Sattarivand and colleagues[23] presented an alternative algorithm. In 2005, Du and colleagues[24] described a perturbation-based method for calculating the matrix coefficients for the GTM method.[21] This technique allows one to take into account the nonlinearity of iterative reconstruction methods. Although developed for single-photon emission CT (SPECT), it is also applicable to PET data.

Voxel-based additive and multiplicative methods (B)

In previous methods, the outcome was a corrected regional mean value; but in 1988, Videen and colleagues[25] proposed a PVC method for voxel-by-voxel correction. A single VOI was used, and RC values were determined for each voxel within the VOI. The application was neurology, and a VOI corresponding to brain tissue was obtained by segmentation of a CT image. It corrected for spill-out but not for spill-in, assuming no background activity. Meltzer and colleagues[26] implemented this method, using MR imaging instead of CT images. Müller-Gärtner and colleagues[27] developed this method further by introducing a spill-in correction term. The brain was segmented into gray matter (GM), white matter (WM), and cerebrospinal fluid (CSF); the correction was applied to GM voxels only, including correction for spill-in from WM, assuming the true mean value in WM could be directly estimated. Erlandsson and colleagues[28] proposed a method, combining the GTM technique for estimation of the VOI mean values, with a Müller-Gärtner–type approach for performing a voxel-based correction of each VOI. With this method, called multi-target correction (MTC), the entire image could be corrected on a voxel-by-voxel basis and no prior information was required.

Purely multiplicative methods (C)

In 1984, Kessler and colleagues[29] extended the RC method in order to take into account spill-in from activity in the background. Correction factors were determined for given target-to-background ratios, which simultaneously corrected for spill-in and spill-out. In order to find the right RC value to use, it is necessary to know the lesion size and the target-to-background ratio. Gallivanone and colleagues[30] proposed methods to determine this information directly from PVE-affected PET images. In 1996, Yang and colleagues[31] presented a voxel-based method for neurology. This method

is a purely multiplicative method, which is applied to the entire image. The brain was segmented into GM, WM, and CSF; an assumption had to be made regarding the relative activity concentrations in the 3 regions. In 2011, Thomas and colleagues[16] presented a method called region-based voxel-wise correction (RBV), similar to MTC,[28] in which the GTM method[21] was combined with the voxel-based correction approach by Yang and colleagues.[31] Erlandsson and colleagues[1] proposed an alternative algorithm, called iterative Yang (iY), in which the first step of RBV was replaced by an iterative procedure for estimation of the regional mean values, avoiding the GTM step.

Wavelet-transform methods (D)

In 2006, Boussion and colleagues[32] presented a novel approach for PVC, in which details from a high-resolution anatomic image were integrated into a low-resolution PET (or SPECT) image in the wavelet domain. Wavelet coefficients from the anatomic image, corresponding to high spatial frequencies, were transferred to the PET image, after scaling by the ratio of the wavelet coefficients from the two images at a lower frequency. Shidahara and colleagues[33] presented an improved version of this method, in which the anatomic image was first segmented and parcellated using an anatomic atlas. When the method was evaluated using simulated dynamic PET data, the results showed improved quantification[34]; when applied to real clinical data, the results were comparable with those of the GTM method.[35]

Deconvolution methods (E)

In 2010, Segobin and colleagues[36] presented an iterative deconvolution algorithm, combined with regional averaging based on a partially segmented anatomic image. This approach could be useful when reliable segmentation was possible for only part of the image. Bousse and colleagues[37] proposed a postreconstruction deconvolution technique, based on a maximum penalized likelihood algorithm, whereby the PET image is described by a model, assuming the existence of activity classes that behave like hidden Markov random fields, driven by a segmented MR image. The method outperformed other postreconstruction PVC methods when the segmented MR imaging was inconsistent with the PET image.

Segmentation-free methods (F)

In 2012, Wang and Fei[38] proposed a PVC method based on iterative deconvolution within a bayesian framework, which included an edge-preserving smoothness constraint. The constraint was imposed using a neighborhood structure, including voxels depending primarily on the difference in PET image values and secondly on the difference in MR imaging values. Yan and colleagues[39] also proposed a novel postreconstruction method, which did not require segmentation of the MR image. It was based on the assumption that a linear relationship exists between PET and MR imaging intensities in a local neighborhood around each voxel.

Reconstruction-Based Methods

Anatomic data can be incorporated into an iterative image reconstruction method as a priori information (or just prior) within a bayesian framework. As a result, the reconstruction algorithm is guided toward solutions, which have higher probability of being correct, which is known as a maximum a posteriori (MAP) algorithm. An alternative is to use penalized likelihood algorithms, although, in practice, the two approaches are quite similar. Traditionally, a smoothing prior would be used in order to limit the noise amplification, often seen in iterative algorithms. However, this also results in resolution degradation. The role of the anatomic prior is to restrict the resolution degradation and preserve anatomic features in the image. The correction for PVE is achieved by modeling the PSF during the reconstruction process. We can distinguish between different types of prior: some use the spatial distribution of the anatomic image and some the image intensity.

Spatial prior methods (G)
In 1991, Chen and colleagues[40] presented a bayesian reconstruction algorithm, incorporating anatomic boundary information from CT or MR images. They achieved significant improvement in image quality with simulated data. Fessler and colleagues[41] propose a penalized likelihood reconstruction method with boundary information from MR images, which took into account possible errors in the boundary information due to errors in the coregistration or segmentation. This effect was achieved by blurring the corresponding weights in the penalty term. Gindi and colleagues[42] proposed a bayesian reconstruction method, which used an edge map from an anatomic image, taking into account the uncertainty in the location of the edges by a spatially varying modulation of the probability. Ouyang and colleagues[43] presented a bayesian reconstruction algorithm based on the joint probability of structural and functional boundaries. Boundary information was extracted from anatomic images, but only those boundaries that had high joint probability with the corresponding PET data were used. Chiao and colleagues[44] presented a penalized

likelihood reconstruction algorithm with anatomic boundary information for cardiac perfusion studies, with coregistration parameters included in the optimization process.

In 1996, Ardekani and colleagues[45] proposed an anatomically guided reconstruction algorithm that did not require segmentation of the MR image. It was based on the cross-entropy between the estimated PET image and a prior image model, obtained by edge-preserving smoothing of the previous estimate. The weights of the smoothing kernel were determined for each voxel, based on the difference in the MR image values. Bowsher and colleagues[46] presented a bayesian algorithm for reconstructing PET or SPECT images and, at the same time, segmenting them into several regions. Anatomic information was used by assigning higher prior probabilities to segmentations in which each segmented region stayed within a single anatomic region. Lipinski and colleagues[47] presented a bayesian reconstruction method, which assumed that all voxels within an anatomic region have values belonging to a Gaussian distribution with a given mean value. The method resulted in images with low noise but was sensitive to incomplete or erroneous anatomic information. Sastry and Carson[48] proposed a similar algorithm in which a Gaussian distribution was assumed for different tissue types (GM, WM, CSF, and *other*). Each voxel was modeled as being composed of the different tissue types in proportions determined by a segmented MR image. Furthermore, a smoothness constraint was used for each separate tissue type.

In 2002, Comtat and colleagues[49] presented a modified version of the algorithm proposed by Fessler and colleagues,[41] in which the anatomic labels were blurred in order to take into account possible registration errors. Baete and colleagues[50] presented a MAP algorithm for fludeoxyglucose (FDG) brain studies. The MR images were segmented into fuzzy classes corresponding to GM, WM, CSF, and *other*. For the purpose of calculating spill-in to the GM region, the WM and CSF regions were assumed to be uniform. Bowsher and colleagues[51] proposed a segmentation-free approach for incorporating MR imaging information into the reconstruction process, similar to the one proposed by Ardekani and colleagues.[45] An edge-preserving smoothing operation was used. The smoothing kernel was generated by choosing a subset of voxels within a neighborhood, with the smallest difference in MR imaging values. In 2010, Vunckx and Nuyts[52] described an improved version of this prior, which takes into account the fact that the voxel neighborhoods selected are not symmetric.

Intensity prior methods (H)

In 2000, Rangarajan and colleagues[53] introduced a novel bayesian framework for incorporating anatomic information into emission tomographic reconstruction, which did not require that the anatomic and functional regions were exactly homologous. The algorithm used a prior based on the mutual information, calculated from the joint histogram for the two images. A segmented anatomic image was used. In 2005, Somayajula and colleagues[54] presented a segmentation-free algorithm, based on the mutual information between various image features in the PET and anatomic images. The algorithm was sensitive to local maxima, and it was necessary to start with a good initial estimate. Nuyts[55] compared 2 anatomically driven MAP reconstruction algorithms with priors based on mutual information and joint entropy of the image intensities, respectively. He found that the joint entropy prior was superior, although local maxima could lead to convergence problems. Tang and Rahmim[56] also developed a MAP reconstruction algorithm, with a joint entropy prior. Using simulated data, they obtained improved noise versus bias tradeoff even in a lesion in the PET image, which had no anatomic correspondence.

In 2010, Tang and colleagues[57] presented a method, which incorporated anatomic information into an algorithm for direct reconstruction of parametric images from dynamic PET data. The method was based on a graphical analysis approach,[58] and the anatomic information was incorporated using a joint entropy prior within a MAP algorithm. Pedemonte and colleagues[59] presented a MAP reconstruction algorithm with a prior based on class conditional joint entropy in order to take into account the underlying tissue composition. The MR imaging was assumed to be composed of GM, WM, CSF, and *other* with Gaussian-distributed image intensities. The method outperformed conventional methods based on joint entropy. Somayajula and colleagues[60] described an approach with priors based on mutual information and joint entropy. Scale-space theory provided a framework for the analysis of images at different levels of detail and presented a solution to the nonspatial nature of these measures. The scale-space features were defined as the original image, the image blurred at different scales, and the Laplacians of the blurred images. In 2015, Tang and Rahmim[61] developed a MAP reconstruction algorithm with a joint entropy prior in which local spatial information was incorporated using a wavelet decomposition. The algorithm performed better than a standard joint entropy MAP algorithm, based on image intensity only, in the case of noisy data.

Diffusion prior methods (I)

In 2009, Chan and colleagues[62] explored an alternative approach to incorporating an anatomic prior into PET image reconstruction, in particular for the situation whereby lesions are apparent in the emission images but not in the corresponding anatomic images. The proposed method was based on an anatomically adaptive anisotropic median-diffusion filtering prior. The proposed prior could yield improved lesion contrast and reduced bias without requiring knowledge of lesion outlines. Kazantsev and colleagues[63] proposed a penalized maximum-likelihood algorithm, incorporating an anatomically driven anisotropic diffusion filter, with edge-preserving denoising characteristics, which has the ability to retain information that was absent in the anatomic image.

A level set method (J)

In 2011, Cheng-Liao and Qi[64] proposed an approach to MAP reconstruction of PET images with a level set prior guided by anatomic edges, which did not assume an exact match between PET and anatomic boundaries but encouraged similarity between the two.

CLINICAL APPLICATIONS OF PARTIAL VOLUME CORRECTION

PET/MR imaging offers clear advantages for PVC. The ability to acquire anatomic information sequentially or even simultaneously to the acquisition of PET data helps alleviate many of the image registration issues that can be problematic with these correction techniques. Furthermore, the exquisite level of soft tissue contrast offers advantages to CT when it comes to feature definition and can also give a better understanding of the tissue mix in PET voxels. The recent introduction of PET/MR as an imaging modality means that there is a dearth of literature on clinical PVC on these scanners. The techniques discussed in the following section describe the application of partial volume methodologies to clinical PET data. Most of the methods described can be applied to PET/MR data and also give an appreciation of the challenges that will be faced when applying such techniques to PET/MR studies.

Cardiology

In nuclear cardiology, there is a clear need for PVC, although it is not commonly applied in clinical practice. For the assessment of myocardial blood flow, uptake of tracer is measured in tissue, which has a thickness of around 15 mm in its systolic phase and typically becomes much thinner in the diastolic phase. The resulting changes in partial volume losses can be visualized when viewing electrocardiogram (ECG)-gated PET data. Apparent changes in blood flow are seen throughout the cardiac cycle, when in reality, for most patients the blood flow should be relatively stable. The problem becomes more of an issue when we also consider the radionuclides typically used for myocardial perfusion imaging in PET. Nitrogen 13–ammonia, oxygen 15 (^{15}O)–water, and rubidium 82 (^{82}Rb)–chloride are 3 agents commonly used in myocardial perfusion imaging, with each emitting more energetic positrons than the frequently used fluorine 18 (^{18}F). Indeed ^{82}Rb emits very energetic positrons, which, because of the longer positron path, lead to poorer spatial resolution than that typically seen in PET. The correction for changes in apparent blood flow across the cardiac cycle and the relative difference between ^{18}F and ^{82}Rb PET has been assessed in an article by Johnson and colleagues.[65] To correct for the change in PVEs, the investigators follow a 2-step approach. In the first step, the change in apparent uptake at end diastole compared with end systole is assessed to calculate the relative difference in PVEs at the two phases. Then using phantom data with known thicknesses and partial volume losses, the correction for end systole is determined; from this the correction for end diastole is derived. Using the ECG-gated data to determine the amount of time spent in the diastolic and systolic phases, it is then possible to obtain average whole heart cycle PVC factors for ungated images.

The assessment of uptake in the myocardial tissue is not the only issue in myocardial perfusion imaging. Proper quantitative analysis of perfusion requires the use of kinetic modeling, which brings its own associated problems: the losses/spill-out of myocardial uptake into the surrounding areas, including the ventricular cavities, and spill-in of activity into the myocardium from the ventricular cavities. Although the latter is not too problematic at late time phases where blood pool activity is limited, at early and intermediate dynamic time frames, there can be significant activity in the blood pool and low but growing activity in the myocardium. This problem can be complicated further as a VOI in the ventricular cavity may be used as an image-derived input function for the kinetic modeling. One of the earliest PVC methods for myocardial imaging, suggested by Herrero and colleagues,[66] assumes a Gaussian point spread function representation of spatial resolution can be convolved with image data of known dimensions to estimate partial volume losses. The investigators used a previously calculated value of the point spread function, an assumed

thickness of myocardium, and carbon 11 (^{11}C)–monoxide PET as a way of measuring the size of the ventricular cavity to calculate the partial volume losses in a series of dog studies. In a study by Iida and colleagues,[67] 2 methods of PVC were evaluated for the correction of myocardial perfusion data. The first measurement involved the inclusion of a tissue fraction in the kinetic model of ^{15}O-water data, whereas the other method used a combination of transmission scan imaging and ^{11}C-monoxide imaging to produce images of extravascular density. Of course, these techniques are applied to dynamic data, with no regard given to the differences across the cardiac cycle.

In recent years there has been a plethora of software available to calculate myocardial blood flow,[68] with several different methods used to deal with PVEs. Some of these solutions take a simple approach to minimize PVEs by assuming fixed global values of partial volume loss and by using image-derived input function volumes placed in positions with minimal spill-in effects from surrounding tissue. Other researchers have used generalized factor analysis of the dynamic data itself in an attempt to intrinsically correct for PVEs.[69] An alternative approach that has become popular in commercialized software[70,71] is that proposed by Hutchins and colleagues[72] in 1990. It assumes that if the blood to myocardium spillover plus the tissue blood-fraction is equal to f_b, then the myocardial activity contribution can be represented by $1-f_b$. This parameter can then be incorporated into the kinetic models to determine partial volume corrected kinetic parameters. This technique has since been modified further by using whole myocardium VOIs to reduce the spillover effects into the image-derived input function, which are in turn used to derive better regional values of myocardial blood flow.[73]

Oncology

In oncology, the application of partial volume techniques in clinical use is more limited. In the most part, clinics report uptake in terms of maximum pixel value rather than the mean value in a region/tumor in an attempt to minimize the issues of partial volume losses. Of course, this is a primitive and rather limited solution because the region/tumor uptake is already likely to be affected by PVEs if it is small in size and the reliance of a single maximum voxel value is also not robust. The introduction of standardized uptake value (SUV) peak, which looks at uptake in a group of pixels, helps overcome the robustness to noise issues but can still be affected by partial volume issues. There are also other issues to consider when introducing PVC in oncology. Is correction required for a tumor volume or for an image? Will the VOI be defined on the PET or corresponding anatomic image? Can the technique be easily applied and used in a busy PET clinic?

By the far the most common form of PVC performed in oncology PET is the use of recovery coefficients. Assuming tumors are spherical and that their diameters can be determined, these methods use phantom measurements to predict the underestimation of uptake due to spill-out and any spill-in of surrounding tissues. Adler and colleagues[74] were early proponents of this method in the imaging of lymph nodes in breast imaging although spill-in effects were not considered. Avril and colleagues[75–77] expanded this method, again in breast cancer, to look at different contrasts in phantoms and was, thus, indirectly looking at spill-in effects. Since these early attempts, further refinements have been made. Vesselle and colleagues[78] working in lung cancer introduced a background region into the correction to deal with spill-in effects, something that is particularly important for small tumors. This approach was developed further by Hickeson and colleagues[79] who used very specific concentric background VOIs and Hofheinz and colleagues[80] who developed a yet more complex method for background region-of-interest (ROI) determination. The Hofheinz technique has also been introduced into a clinical software platform to create a simple and automated approach to oncological PVC with improved intraoperator and interoperator error.[81] Salavati and colleagues[82] applied this technique to FDG PET/CT studies of lung lesions with and without respiratory gating. They found that after PVC, the SUV_{mean} increased substantially and that the PVE seemed to be the dominant source of quantitative error of lung malignancies. However, they found no clinically significant difference between respiratory-gated and nongated data after PVC.

When applying such PVCs, these and other investigators have found improvements in diagnostic performance or better correlation with other physiologic metrics. The success of the RC technique is based on its simplicity, although it does have its limitations. The assumptions that the tumor is spherical and that its uptake is homogeneous are questionable, particularly for larger tumors that may also have necrotic centers. Another issue is the determination of the tumor radius. The higher-spatial-resolution CT component from PET/CT or indeed the MR imaging component from PET/MR imaging systems can potentially help, but unfortunately the metabolic volume does not always correspond to the anatomic volumes that these modalities offer. Defining tumor volumes based on PET has been attempted,[79,83] but the robustness of this technique has yet to be proven particularly in smaller lower-contrast lesions. A final issue with RC techniques is that the correction is performed on a volume and not on the image as a whole. This issue is generally not a problem in oncological PET whereby the tumor uptake is typically the main output metric of interest, but this approach is not helpful when the general distribution of uptake or heterogeneity of uptake within a tumor is required.

Other partial volume techniques in oncological PET are more complex and because of this only appear in proof-of-concept studies with small patient numbers.[32,84,85] An approach that has gained some interest is the use of deconvolution using the Van Cittert[2] or Lucy-Richardson techniques[86] to iteratively recover resolution losses across an image. One problem with these methods is that noise can be amplified using these approaches, although denoising using, for example, a wavelet methodology has been applied with good results.[86,87] Another issue with deconvolution techniques is that they depend on an accurate measurement of spatial resolution (point-spread function). Because spatial resolution changes across the PET field of view, this can be difficult to model. This issue affects other PVC methods as well, but it is more critical for deconvolution techniques, as no other information is used.

The wide choice of PVC algorithms leads to difficulty in choosing the most appropriate algorithm for oncological imaging. In PET, although accuracy is important, because many patients are assessed longitudinally for treatment response and/or disease progression, test-retest reproducibility is equally important. Hoetjes and colleagues[83] evaluated 3 approaches of PVC for accuracy and reproducibility in simulated and patient data. The study compared an iterative deconvolution approach, correction as part of iterative reconstruction, and a mask-based approach and found reconstruction-based PVC performed best, although each of the other two approaches were adequate and easy-to-implement alternatives. Of course, it is assumed that PVC provides improved quantitative performance. Although this may be the case, it does not necessarily lead to improved diagnostic outcomes.[87,88]

Neurology

In PET, the widest use of PVC techniques is seen in neurologic applications. The size and thickness of the areas of interest in the brain together with the relative ease of image segmentation and image registration have led to a plethora of literature describing various methodologies and their clinical application. Since its initial conception and application in ^{11}C-carfentanil PET by Meltzer and colleagues,[26] a simple segmentation approach of dealing with atrophy-related signal losses has been popular. Ibáñez and colleagues[89] used the method to show that hypometabolism as seen in FDG PET is a real phenomenon and not something caused by cortical atrophy-related signal loss. Following on from this, Meltzer and colleagues[90] and Ibáñez and colleagues[91] using the same technique also found that apparent reductions in cortical glucose metabolism with increasing age were not real but actually caused by normal age-related increases in cortical atrophy. Refinements to the Meltzer technique have also been developed. Adapting the approach to include a spatially variant PSF, Labbé and colleagues[92] applied their technique in the analysis of 4 control and 8 patients with Alzheimer disease imaged using ^{18}F-FDG PET. However, the most popular variant of the original Meltzer method, which replaced a single brain tissue compartment with individual GM and WM compartments, was that proposed by Müller-Gärtner and colleagues.[27] Giovacchini and colleagues,[93] using dynamic imaging of 8 young and 7 old subjects, confirmed with the application of both Meltzer and Müller-Gärtner methods that blood flow was not affected by healthy aging. Conversely, looking at a different biomarker, Bencherif and colleagues,[94] imaging 14 healthy control subjects with ^{11}C-carfentanil, showed an age effect in uptake with PVC, which disappeared when no correction was applied. In turn, the Müller-Gärtner method has also seen slight revisions,[95] which have been applied in an FDG PET aging study.[96] The relative advantages of 2 (Meltzer) or 3 (Müller-Gärtner) segmentations have also been explored.[97] Although 3 segmented compartments lead to slightly higher accuracy, they can be less robust than 2 compartments because of the misregistration and segmentation errors that can prove problematic for these techniques.

There are also other PVC techniques that have been applied to clinical data. Goffin and colleagues[98] found benefits in applying anatomic-based prior MAP reconstructions to reduce PVEs when trying to localize focal cortical dysplasias in epileptic patients imaged with FDG. While in the area of Alzheimer disease, Thomas and colleagues[16] compared the Van-Cittert and RBV method together with the Müller-Gärtner method in a series of 70 amyloid PET scans, with the RBV method performing best out of the 3 methods. Another commonly used method of PVC in neurologic PET is the GTM method.[21] In 2008, Rousset and colleagues[99] applied this method to 90 ^{11}C-raclopride studies of healthy volunteers, showing increased and also less heterogeneous uptake (in terms of caudate vs putamen) when compared with uncorrected studies.

The application of PVC techniques is becoming more widely reported in clinical dementia populations, whereby atrophy is clearly a common issue. Drzezga and colleagues[100] used commercialized Müller-Gärtner PVC software for correction of ^{11}C-labelled Pittsburgh compound B (PIB) and FDG studies of patients with Alzheimer disease and semantic dementia. The same group also used the technique in a longitudinal study of 15 patients, again with ^{11}C-PIB and FDG in an attempt to follow the changes in Alzheimer disease over a period of 2 years.[101] Further longitudinal amyloid PET studies by Su and colleagues[102] with the GTM method and Meltzer method and Brendel and colleagues[103] using just the GTM method have also recommended the use of PVC in these types of studies, with the GTM providing slightly better results than the Meltzer method.

Once more, one of the concerns with applying these techniques in longitudinal studies is the test-retest reproducibility of these methods with issues typically arising from errors in image registration and segmentation. In the study by Su and colleagues,[102] segmentation errors led to test-retest variability of around 1.5%, which compared well with the 2% errors from the VOIs used to derive regional uptake. However, it would seem that the use of different segmentation algorithms can lead to different results in the same patients, suggesting that segmentation algorithms are not interchangeable when performing PVC.[9,10] Nevertheless, the recent swell in the use of PVC in dementia PET studies suggests that PVC may become mainstream in these studies. See **Box 3** for a clinical example.

Box 3
Clinical example: neurology

Fig. 5 shows images from a clinical study on a patient with semantic dementia and left temporal lobe atrophy. PET studies were performed with 2 different tracers: ^{18}F-FDG for glucose metabolism and the amyloid tracer ^{18}F-AV45. Images are shown without PVC and with PVC using the iY method.[1] The 2 tracers have different distributions. The AV45 scan was amyloid negative, with mainly nonspecific uptake in WM, whereas the FDG study shows mainly uptake in GM.

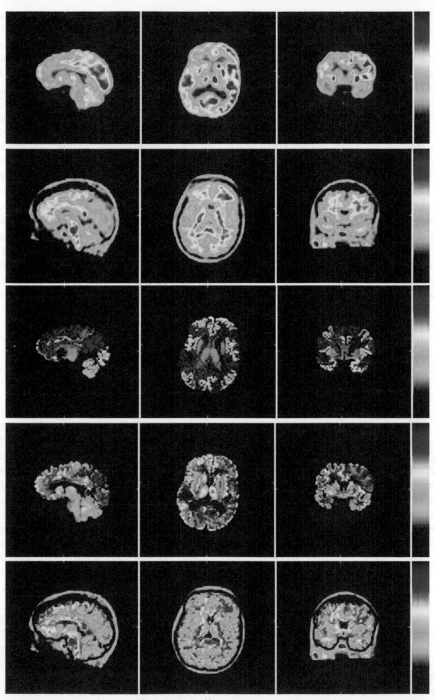

Fig. 5. Data from a clinical study with ^{18}F-FDG and ^{18}F-AV45 on the same patient, including uncorrected FDG study (*first row*), uncorrected AV45 study (*second row*), segmented/parcellated MR imaging scan (*third row*), corrected FDG study (*fourth row*), and corrected AV45 study (*fifth row*), with sagittal (*left column*), transaxial (*middle column*), and coronal (*right column*) sections. Each image volume was normalized independently.

Vascular

Beyond the derivation of corrected image-derived input functions in vessels,[104] there have also been studies looking at correcting uptake in features

within the vessel itself. Izquierdo-Garcia and colleagues[105] used a GTM methodology to correct uptake in plaques in 7 patients imaged with FDG and found corrected data to be both accurate and reproducible in the carotid artery wall. Reeps and colleagues[106] looked at performing PVC in abdominal aortic aneurysms in 23 patients undergoing FDG PET imaging. Using a novel approach that created a geometric model of the area of interest, and a factor that accounted for the spatial resolution of the PET system, the study found that PVC was not mandatory for such imaging but may provide a role in helping to stratify patients. Burg and colleagues[107] compared various methods for quantifying tracer uptake in the aortic vascular wall in [18]FDG PET studies using simulations based on an anthropomorphic digital phantom. They found that PVC using the GTM method gave the most reproducible results, although some bias remained because of the low dimensions of the vascular wall. Blomberg and colleagues[108] evaluated the impact of a novel PVC method, based on contrast-enhanced CT data, on the quantification of arterial wall ^{18}F-FDG uptake. The PVC method used was similar in principle to the Hofheinz method.[80] Their study showed that PVC significantly influences quantification of arterial wall ^{18}F-FDG uptake. On the other hand, they also found a good correlation between the values before and after PVC at 180 minutes after injection and concluded that the uncorrected values could be used as a measure of arterial ^{18}F-FDG uptake.[108]

DISCUSSION

There is increasing evidence that PVC is necessary in order to guarantee quantitative accuracy in emission tomography, but there is reluctance to apply PVC routinely in clinical practice where there continues to be reliance on visual interpretation for many routine studies. There continues to be uncertainty by many clinicians regarding the method of choice, and the absence of widely accepted and validated commercial software does little to encourage more widespread use. There also continues to be concern regarding the various potential sources of error (eg, Frouin and colleagues[8]). Most PVC methods rely on having accurately registered anatomic data (preferably MR imaging), but the lack of ready availability of these data and historical problems with cross-vendor compatibility have been barriers to routine use; the availability of PET/MR imaging systems certainly removes (or at least reduces) these barriers. As mentioned earlier, registration is not entirely guaranteed with PET/MR imaging; but the degree of misregistration is certainly reduced, and nonrigid registration is unlikely to be needed. Of course the underlying assumption in many PVC methods is that the anatomic edge information matches the tissue boundaries underlying the functional or molecular image, which is not necessarily the case (eg, there may be cellular invasion of tissues not visible in the anatomic image). Note also that nonrigid registration between high-resolution MR imaging and the limited-resolution PET can attempt to align identified edges in a way that invalidates the PVC procedure. There are similar concerns regarding segmentation approaches that are often necessary, especially where structures are very small (eg, blood vessels). A small error in segmentation may represent a sizable percentage error in estimated volume and, hence, a significant source of error. Approaches that avoid the need for segmentation may be preferred, for example, techniques that use local variation in MR contrast directly.[39,45,51]

In some cases it can be argued that PVC makes little difference to interpretation or indeed can have a negative influence due to enhanced noise. However, in situations when volume is changing in serial studies, misinterpretation is very common. Also if activity distribution changes in time, as is clearly the case in kinetic studies, there can be significant errors introduced by PVEs. Take the example of a dynamic cardiac study whereby activity is initially circulating in the blood with significant spillover to the myocardium but later may be concentrated in the myocardium itself. Variation in the spillover will clearly affect the resulting time activity curves for both the ventricle (and image-derived input function) and myocardium, affecting any derived kinetic parameters. A recent article by Su and colleagues[102] highlights the importance of performing PVC in kinetic amyloid studies, which are being used to further elucidate uptake patterns in patients with dementia. Other groups have also shown the importance of PVC for kinetic analysis.[8,109,110] PVC is also important for accurate estimation of image-derived input functions.[111] Further information on this topic can be found in Ref.[104]

An aspect of PVC less commonly addressed is the influence of the tissue fraction effect; in general this accounts for the uptake of tracer in selected targets contained within a voxel (eg, uptake in the cellular matrix rather than blood or air in the lung). In fact heterogeneous uptake of tracer is invariably the case within the volume of tissue contained in a typical image voxel. Kinetic analysis often does take into account a vascular component, but again problems arise if the nontarget tissue fraction varies spatially or temporally. Research on methods to tackle this problem, specifically applicable to lung studies, has been published (Lambrou and colleagues,[112] Holman and colleagues[113]). This work relies on identifying air fraction from CT density and/or blood fraction based on kinetic analysis as a basis for deriving tissue fraction corrected values, which may provide better indices of the underlying mechanism of uptake in disease or treatment response during therapy.

There is a distinct shortage of published work on the direct comparison of different PVC methods. Validation is not a trivial exercise as it requires ground truth knowledge of tracer distribution, which is not possible in vivo. Comparison of discrimination power is commonly used to justify the choice of individual methods, although in practice the effect can be small (eg, Thomas and colleagues[16]). The alternative approach is based on simulation. The challenge is to implement simulation methods that are clinically realistic, that use analysis techniques that are independent of the methods used for PVC, and that provide meaningful metrics for comparative purposes. Ideally test datasets should be made openly available so that PVC can be tested by individual developers, in much the same way as the clinical datasets made available for evaluation through Alzheimer's Disease Neuroimaging Initiative.[114] Development of such a library has been the aim of work undertaken in conjunction with the European Union Cooperation in Science and Technology (EU COST) project (TD1007) with suggested approaches and preliminary results published by Hutton and colleagues[115] and Thomas and colleagues.[116]

ACKNOWLEDGMENTS

The authors would like to thank Dr Jonathan Schott, Dementia Research Unit, University College London for providing the clinical brain data included.

REFERENCES

1. Erlandsson K, Buvat I, Pretorius PH, et al. A review of partial volume correction techniques for emission tomography and their applications in neurology, cardiology and oncology. Phys Med Biol 2012;57:R119–59.
2. Teo BK, Seo Y, Bacharach SL, et al. Partial-volume correction in PET: validation of an iterative postreconstruction method with phantom and patient data. J Nucl Med 2007;48:802–10.
3. Tohka J, Reilhac A. Deconvolution-based partial volume correction in Raclopride-PET and Monte Carlo comparison to MR-based method. Neuroimage 2008;39:1570–84.
4. Reader AJ, Julyan PJ, Williams H, et al. EM algorithm system modeling by image-space techniques for PET reconstruction. IEEE Trans Nucl Sci 2003; 50:1392–7.
5. Alessio AM, Kinahan PE, Lewellen TK. Modeling and incorporation of system response functions in 3-D whole body PET. IEEE Trans Med Imaging 2006;25:828–37.
6. Rousset O, Rahmim A, Alavi A, et al. Partial volume correction strategies in PET. PET Clin 2007; 2:235–49.
7. Bettinardi V, Castiglioni I, De Bernardi E, et al. PET quantification: strategies for partial volume correction. Clin Transl Imaging 2014;2:199–218.
8. Frouin V, Comtat C, Reilhac A, et al. Correction of partial-volume effect for PET striatal imaging: fast implementation and study of robustness. J Nucl Med 2002;43:1715–26.
9. Zaidi H, Ruest T, Schoenahl F, et al. Comparative assessment of statistical brain MR image segmentation algorithms and their impact on partial volume correction in PET. Neuroimage 2006;32:1591–607.
10. Gutierrez D, Montandon ML, Assal F, et al. Anatomically guided voxel-based partial volume effect correction in brain PET: impact of MRI segmentation. Comput Med Imaging Graph 2012;36:610–9.
11. Hutton BF, Braun M, Slomka P. Image registration techniques in nuclear medicine imaging. In: Zaidi H, editor. Quantitative analysis in nuclear Medicine imaging. Berlin: Springer; 2006. p. 272–307.
12. Slomka PJ, Baum RP. Multimodality image registration with software: state-of-the-art. Eur J Nucl Med Mol Imaging 2009;36(Suppl 1):S44–55.
13. Klein A, Andersson J, Ardekani BA, et al. Evaluation of 14 nonlinear deformation algorithms applied to human brain MRI registration. Neuroimage 2009; 46:786–802.
14. Townsend DW. Multimodality imaging of structure and function. Phys Med Biol 2008;53:R1–39.
15. Pichler BJ, Kolb A, Nagele T, et al. PET/MRI: paving the way for the next generation of clinical multimodality imaging applications. J Nucl Med 2010;51:333–6.
16. Thomas BA, Erlandsson K, Modat M, et al. The importance of appropriate partial volume correction for PET quantification in Alzheimer's disease. Eur J Nucl Med Mol Imaging 2011;38:1104–19.
17. Nuyts J, Baete K, Beque D, et al. Comparison between MAP and postprocessed ML for image reconstruction in emission tomography when anatomical knowledge is available. IEEE Trans Med Imaging 2005;24:667–75.
18. Hoffman EJ, Huang SC, Phelps ME. Quantitation in positron emission computed tomography: 1. effect of object size. J Comput Assist Tomogr 1979;3: 299–308.
19. Soret M, Bacharach SL, Buvat I. Partial-volume effect in PET tumor imaging. J Nucl Med 2007;48:932–45.
20. Henze E, Huang SC, Ratib O, et al. Measurements of regional tissue and blood-pool radiotracer concentrations from serial tomographic images of the heart. J Nucl Med 1983;24:987–96.

21. Rousset OG, Ma Y, Evans AC. Correction for partial volume effects in PET: principle and validation. J Nucl Med 1998;39:904–11.

22. Labbé C, Koepp MJ, Ashburner J, et al. Absolute PET quantification with correction for partial volume effects within cerebral structures. In: Carson RE, Daube-Witherspoon ME, Herscovitch P, editors. Quantitative functional brain imaging with positron emission tomography. San Diego (CA): Academic Press; 1998. p. 59–66.

23. Sattarivand M, Kusano M, Poon I, et al. Symmetric geometric transfer matrix partial volume correction for PET imaging: principle, validation and robustness. Phys Med Biol 2012;57:7101–16.

24. Du Y, Tsui BM, Frey EC. Partial volume effect compensation for quantitative brain SPECT imaging. IEEE Trans Med Imaging 2005;24:969–76.

25. Videen TO, Perlmutter JS, Mintun MA, et al. Regional correction of positron emission tomography data for the effects of cerebral atrophy. J Cereb Blood Flow Metab 1988;8:662–70.

26. Meltzer CC, Leal JP, Mayberg HS, et al. Correction of PET data for partial volume effects in human cerebral cortex by MR imaging. J Comput Assist Tomogr 1990;14:561–70.

27. Müller-Gärtner HW, Links JM, Prince JL, et al. Measurement of radiotracer concentration in brain gray matter using positron emission tomography: MRI-based correction for partial volume effects. J Cereb Blood Flow Metab 1992;12:571–83.

28. Erlandsson K, Wong AT, van Heertum R, et al. An improved method for voxel-based partial volume correction in PET and SPECT. Neuroimage 2006;31:T84.

29. Kessler RM, Ellis JR Jr, Eden M. Analysis of emission tomographic scan data: limitations imposed by resolution and background. J Comput Assist Tomogr 1984;8:514–22.

30. Gallivanone F, Stefano A, Grosso E, et al. PVE correction in PET-CT whole-body oncological studies from PVE-affected images. IEEE Trans Nucl Sci 2011;58:736–47.

31. Yang J, Huang SC, Mega M, et al. Investigation of partial volume correction methods for brain FDG PET studies. IEEE Trans Nucl Sci 1996;43:3322–7.

32. Boussion N, Hatt M, Lamare F, et al. A multiresolution image based approach for correction of partial volume effects in emission tomography. Phys Med Biol 2006;51:1857–76.

33. Shidahara M, Tsoumpas C, Hammers A, et al. Functional and structural synergy for resolution recovery and partial volume correction in brain PET. Neuroimage 2009;44:340–8.

34. Shidahara M, Tsoumpas C, McGinnity CJ, et al. Wavelet-based resolution recovery using an anatomical prior provides quantitative recovery

35. Kim E, Shidahara M, Tsoumpas C, et al. Partial volume correction using structural-functional synergistic resolution recovery: comparison with geometric transfer matrix method. J Cereb Blood Flow Metab 2013;33:914–20.

36. Segobin SH, Matthews JC, Markiewicz PJ, et al. A hybrid between region-based and voxel-based methods for partial volume correction in PET. In: Ziock K, editor. 2010 IEEE nuclear science symposium and medical imaging conference. Knoxville (TN): 2010. p. 3073–8.

37. Bousse A, Pedemonte S, Thomas BA, et al. Markov random field and gaussian mixture for segmented MRI-based partial volume correction in PET. Phys Med Biol 2012;57:6681–705.

38. Wang H, Fei B. An MR image-guided, voxel-based partial volume correction method for PET images. Med Phys 2012;39:179–95.

39. Yan J, Lim JC, Townsend DW. MRI-guided brain PET image filtering and partial volume correction. Phys Med Biol 2015;60:961–76.

40. Chen C-T, Ouyang X, Wong WH, et al. Sensor fusion in image reconstruction. IEEE Trans Nucl Sci 1991;38:687–92.

41. Fessler JA, Clinthorne NH, Rogers WL. Regularized emission image reconstruction using imperfect side information. IEEE Trans Nucl Sci 1992;39:1464–71.

42. Gindi G, Lee M, Rangarajan A, et al. Bayesian reconstruction of functional images using anatomical information as priors. IEEE Trans Med Imaging 1993;12:670–80.

43. Ouyang X, Wong WH, Johnson VE, et al. Incorporation of correlated structural images in PET image reconstruction. IEEE Trans Med Imaging 1994;13:627–40.

44. Chiao PC, Rogers WL, Fessler JA, et al. Model-based estimation with boundary side information or boundary regularization [cardiac emission CT]. IEEE Trans Med Imaging 1994;13:227–34.

45. Ardekani BA, Braun M, Hutton BF, et al. Minimum cross-entropy reconstruction of PET images using prior anatomical information. Phys Med Biol 1996;41:2497–517.

46. Bowsher JE, Johnson VE, Turkington TG, et al. Bayesian reconstruction and use of anatomical a priori information for emission tomography. IEEE Trans Med Imaging 1996;15:673–86.

47. Lipinski B, Herzog H, Rota Kops E, et al. Expectation maximization reconstruction of positron emission tomography images using anatomical magnetic resonance information. IEEE Trans Med Imaging 1997;16:129–36.

48. Sastry S, Carson RE. Multimodality bayesian algorithm for image reconstruction in positron emission

tomography: a tissue composition model. IEEE Trans Med Imaging 1997;16:750–61.

49. Comtat C, Kinahan PE, Fessler JA, et al. Clinically feasible reconstruction of 3D whole-body PET/CT data using blurred anatomical labels. Phys Med Biol 2002;47:1–20.

50. Baete K, Nuyts J, Van Paesschen W, et al. Anatomical-based FDG-PET reconstruction for the detection of hypo-metabolic regions in epilepsy. IEEE Trans Med Imaging 2004;23:510–9.

51. Bowsher JE, Yuan H, Hedlund LW, et al. Utilizing MRI information to estimate F18-FDG distributions in rat flank tumors. In: Seibert JA, editor. IEEE nuclear science symposium and medical imaging conference. vol. 4. Rome (Italy): 2004. p. 2488–92.

52. Vunckx K, Nuyts J. Heuristic modification of an anatomical Markov prior improves its performance. In: Ziock K, editor. 2010 IEEE nuclear science symposium and medical imaging conference. Knoxville (TN): 2010. p. 3262–6.

53. Rangarajan A, Hsiao I-T, Gindi G. A bayesian joint mixture framework for the integration of anatomical information in functional image reconstruction. J Math Imaging Vis 2000;12:199–217.

54. Somayajula S, Asma E, Leahy RM. PET image reconstruction using anatomical information through mutual information based priors. In: Yu B, editor. 2005 IEEE nuclear science symposium and medical imaging conference. vol. 5. Puerto Rico: 2005. p. 2722–6.

55. Nuyts J. The use of mutual information and joint entropy for anatomical priors in emission tomography. In: Yu B, editor. 2007 IEEE nuclear science symposium and medical imaging conference. vol. 6. Honolulu (HI): 2007. p. 4149–54.

56. Tang J, Rahmim A. Bayesian PET image reconstruction incorporating anato-functional joint entropy. Phys Med Biol 2009;54:7063–75.

57. Tang J, Kuwabara H, Wong DF, et al. Direct 4D reconstruction of parametric images incorporating anato-functional joint entropy. Phys Med Biol 2010;55:4261–72.

58. Patlak CS, Blasberg RG. Graphical evaluation of blood-to-brain transfer constants from multiple-time uptake data. Generalizations. J Cereb Blood Flow Metab 1985;5:584–90.

59. Pedemonte S, Cardoso MJ, Bousse A, et al. Class conditional entropic prior for MRI enhanced SPECT reconstruction. In: Ziock K, editor. IEEE nuclear science symposium and medical imaging conference. Knoxville (TN): 2010. p. 3292–300.

60. Somayajula S, Panagiotou C, Rangarajan A, et al. PET image reconstruction using information theoretic anatomical priors. IEEE Trans Med Imaging 2011;30:537–49.

61. Tang J, Rahmim A. Anatomy assisted PET image reconstruction incorporating multi-resolution joint entropy. Phys Med Biol 2015;60:31–48.

62. Chan C, Fulton R, Feng DD, et al. Regularized image reconstruction with an anatomically adaptive prior for positron emission tomography. Phys Med Biol 2009;54:7379–400.

63. Kazantsev D, Arridge SR, Pedemonte S, et al. An anatomically driven anisotropic diffusion filtering method for 3D SPECT reconstruction. Phys Med Biol 2012;57:3793–810.

64. Cheng-Liao J, Qi J. PET image reconstruction with anatomical edge guided level set prior. Phys Med Biol 2011;56:6899–918.

65. Johnson NP, Sdringola S, Gould KL. Partial volume correction incorporating Rb-82 positron range for quantitative myocardial perfusion PET based on systolic-diastolic activity ratios and phantom measurements. J Nucl Cardiol 2011;18:247–58.

66. Herrero P, Markham J, Myears DW, et al. Measurement of myocardial blood flow with positron emission tomography: correction for count spillover and partial volume effects. Math Comput Model 1988;11:807–12.

67. Iida H, Rhodes CG, de Silva R, et al. Myocardial tissue fraction–correction for partial volume effects and measure of tissue viability. J Nucl Med 1991; 32:2169–75.

68. Nesterov SV, Deshayes E, Sciagra R, et al. Quantification of myocardial blood flow in absolute terms using (82)Rb PET imaging: the RUBY-10 Study. JACC Cardiovasc Imaging 2014;7:1119–27.

69. El Fakhri G, Sitek A, Guerin B, et al. Quantitative dynamic cardiac 82Rb PET using generalized factor and compartment analyses. J Nucl Med 2005; 46:1264–71.

70. Klein R, Renaud JM, Ziadi MC, et al. Intra- and inter-operator repeatability of myocardial blood flow and myocardial flow reserve measurements using rubidium-82 PET and a highly automated analysis program. J Nucl Cardiol 2010;17:600–16.

71. Slomka PJ, Alexanderson E, Jacome R, et al. Comparison of clinical tools for measurements of regional stress and rest myocardial blood flow assessed with 13N-ammonia PET/CT. J Nucl Med 2012;53:171–81.

72. Hutchins GD, Schwaiger M, Rosenspire KC, et al. Noninvasive quantification of regional blood flow in the human heart using N-13 ammonia and dynamic positron emission tomographic imaging. J Am Coll Cardiol 1990;15:1032–42.

73. Katoh C, Yoshinaga K, Klein R, et al. Quantification of regional myocardial blood flow estimation with three-dimensional dynamic rubidium-82 PET and modified spillover correction model. J Nucl Cardiol 2012;19:763–74.

74. Adler LP, Crowe JP, al-Kaisi NK, et al. Evaluation of breast masses and axillary lymph nodes with [F-18] 2-deoxy-2-fluoro-D-glucose PET. Radiology 1993;187:743–50.

75. Avril N, Dose J, Janicke F, et al. Metabolic characterization of breast tumors with positron emission tomography using F-18 fluorodeoxyglucose. J Clin Oncol 1996;14:1848–57.

76. Avril N, Bense S, Ziegler SI, et al. Breast imaging with fluorine-18-FDG PET: quantitative image analysis. J Nucl Med 1997;38:1186–91.

77. Avril N, Menzel M, Dose J, et al. Glucose metabolism of breast cancer assessed by 18F-FDG PET: histologic and immunohistochemical tissue analysis. J Nucl Med 2001;42:9–16.

78. Vesselle H, Schmidt RA, Pugsley JM, et al. Lung cancer proliferation correlates with [F-18] fluorodeoxyglucose uptake by positron emission tomography. Clin Cancer Res 2000;6:3837–44.

79. Hickeson M, Yun M, Matthies A, et al. Use of a corrected standardized uptake value based on the lesion size on CT permits accurate characterization of lung nodules on FDG-PET. Eur J Nucl Med Mol Imaging 2002;29:1639–47.

80. Hofheinz F, Langner J, Petr J, et al. A method for model-free partial volume correction in oncological PET. EJNMMI Res 2012;2:16.

81. Torigian DA, Lopez RF, Alapati S, et al. Feasibility and performance of novel software to quantify metabolically active volumes and 3D partial volume corrected SUV and metabolic volumetric products of spinal bone marrow metastases on 18F-FDG-PET/CT. Hell J Nucl Med 2011;14:8–14.

82. Salavati A, Borofsky S, Boon-Keng TK, et al. Application of partial volume effect correction and 4D PET in the quantification of FDG avid lung lesions. Mol Imaging Biol 2015;17:140–8.

83. Hoetjes NJ, van Velden FH, Hoekstra OS, et al. Partial volume correction strategies for quantitative FDG PET in oncology. Eur J Nucl Med Mol Imaging 2010;37:1679–87.

84. Chang G, Chang T, Pan T, et al. Joint correction of respiratory motion artifact and partial volume effect in lung/thoracic PET/CT imaging. Med Phys 2010; 37:6221–32.

85. Barbee DL, Flynn RT, Holden JE, et al. A method for partial volume correction of PET-imaged tumor heterogeneity using expectation maximization with a spatially varying point spread function. Phys Med Biol 2010;55:221–36.

86. Boussion N, Cheze Le Rest C, Hatt M, et al. Incorporation of wavelet-based denoising in iterative deconvolution for partial volume correction in whole-body PET imaging. Eur J Nucl Med Mol Imaging 2009;36:1064–75.

87. Hatt M, Le Pogam A, Visvikis D, et al. Impact of partial-volume effect correction on the predictive and prognostic value of baseline 18F-FDG PET images in esophageal cancer. J Nucl Med 2012;53:12–20.

88. Tsujikawa T, Otsuka H, Morita N, et al. Does partial volume corrected maximum SUV based on count recovery coefficient in 3D-PET/CT correlate with clinical aggressiveness of non-Hodgkin's lymphoma? Ann Nucl Med 2008;22:23–30.

89. Ibáñez V, Pietrini P, Alexander GE, et al. Regional glucose metabolic abnormalities are not the result of atrophy in Alzheimer's disease. Neurology 1998;50:1585–93.

90. Meltzer CC, Cantwell MN, Greer PJ, et al. Does cerebral blood flow decline in healthy aging? A PET study with partial-volume correction. J Nucl Med 2000;41:1842–8.

91. Ibáñez V, Pietrini P, Furey ML, et al. Resting state brain glucose metabolism is not reduced in normotensive healthy men during aging, after correction for brain atrophy. Brain Res Bull 2004;63:147–54.

92. Labbé C, Froment JC, Kennedy A, et al. Positron emission tomography metabolic data corrected for cortical atrophy using magnetic resonance imaging. Alzheimer Dis Assoc Disord 1996;10:141–70.

93. Giovacchini G, Lerner A, Toczek MT, et al. Brain incorporation of 11C-arachidonic acid, blood volume, and blood flow in healthy aging: a study with partial-volume correction. J Nucl Med 2004; 45:1471–9.

94. Bencherif B, Stumpf MJ, Links JM, et al. Application of MRI-based partial-volume correction to the analysis of PET images of mu-opioid receptors using statistical parametric mapping. J Nucl Med 2004;45:402–8.

95. Matsuda H, Ohnishi T, Asada T, et al. Correction for partial-volume effects on brain perfusion SPECT in healthy men. J Nucl Med 2003;44:1243–52.

96. Yanase D, Matsunari I, Yajima K, et al. Brain FDG PET study of normal aging in Japanese: effect of atrophy correction. Eur J Nucl Med Mol Imaging 2005;32:794–805.

97. Meltzer CC, Kinahan PE, Greer PJ, et al. Comparative evaluation of MR-based partial-volume correction schemes for PET. J Nucl Med 1999;40:2053–65.

98. Goffin K, Van Paesschen W, Dupont P, et al. Anatomy-based reconstruction of FDG-PET images with implicit partial volume correction improves detection of hypometabolic regions in patients with epilepsy due to focal cortical dysplasia diagnosed on MRI. Eur J Nucl Med Mol Imaging 2010;37:1148–55.

99. Rousset OG, Collins DL, Rahmim A, et al. Design and implementation of an automated partial volume correction in PET: application to dopamine receptor quantification in the normal human striatum. J Nucl Med 2008;49:1097–106.

100. Drzezga A, Grimmer T, Henriksen G, et al. Imaging of amyloid plaques and cerebral glucose metabolism in semantic dementia and Alzheimer's disease. Neuroimage 2008;39:619–33.

101. Forster S, Yousefi BH, Wester HJ, et al. Quantitative longitudinal interrelationships between brain metabolism and amyloid deposition during a 2-year follow-up in patients with early Alzheimer's disease. Eur J Nucl Med Mol Imaging 2012;39:1927–36.

102. Su Y, Blazey TM, Snyder AZ, et al. Partial volume correction in quantitative amyloid imaging. Neuroimage 2015;107:55–64.

103. Brendel M, Hogenauer M, Delker A, et al. Improved longitudinal [(18)F]-AV45 amyloid PET by white matter reference and VOI-based partial volume effect correction. Neuroimage 2015;108:450–9.

104. Richard MA, Fouquet JP, Lebel R, et al. MR imaging-guided derivation of the input function for PET kinetic modeling PET Clin, in press.

105. Izquierdo-Garcia D, Davies JR, Graves MJ, et al. Comparison of methods for magnetic resonance-guided [18-F]fluorodeoxyglucose positron emission tomography in human carotid arteries: reproducibility, partial volume correction, and correlation between methods. Stroke 2009;40:86–93.

106. Reeps C, Bundschuh RA, Pellisek J, et al. Quantitative assessment of glucose metabolism in the vessel wall of abdominal aortic aneurysms: correlation with histology and role of partial volume correction. Int J Cardiovasc Imaging 2013;29:505–12.

107. Burg S, Dupas A, Stute S, et al. Partial volume effect estimation and correction in the aortic vascular wall in PET imaging. Phys Med Biol 2013;58:7527–42.

108. Blomberg BA, Bashyam A, Ramachandran A, et al. Quantifying [(18)F] fluorodeoxyglucose uptake in the arterial wall: the effects of dual time-point imaging and partial volume effect correction. Eur J Nucl Med Mol Imaging 2015;42:1414–22.

109. Rousset OG, Deep P, Kuwabara H, et al. Effect of partial volume correction on estimates of the influx and cerebral metabolism of 6-[(18)F]fluoro-L-dopa studied with PET in normal control and Parkinson's disease subjects. Synapse 2000;37:81–9.

110. Bowen SL, Byars LG, Michel CJ, et al. Influence of the partial volume correction method on (18)F-fluorodeoxyglucose brain kinetic modelling from dynamic PET images reconstructed with resolution model based OSEM. Phys Med Biol 2013;58:7081–106.

111. Zanotti-Fregonara P, Fadaili el M, Maroy R, et al. Comparison of eight methods for the estimation of the image-derived input function in dynamic [(18)F]-FDG PET human brain studies. J Cereb Blood Flow Metab 2009;29:1825–35.

112. Lambrou T, Groves AM, Erlandsson K, et al. The importance of correction for tissue fraction effects in lung PET: preliminary findings. Eur J Nucl Med Mol Imaging 2011;38:2238–46.

113. Holman BF, Cuplov V, Millner L, et al. Improved correction for the tissue fraction effect in lung PET/CT imaging. Phys Med Biol 2015;60(18):7387–402.

114. Mueller SG, Weiner MW, Thal LJ, et al. Ways toward an early diagnosis in Alzheimer's disease: the Alzheimer's Disease Neuroimaging Initiative (ADNI). Alzheimers Dement 2005;1:55–66.

115. Hutton BF, Thomas BA, Erlandson K, et al. What approach to brain partial volume correction is best for PET/MRI? Nucl Instr Meth A 2013;702:29–33.

116. Thomas BA, Erlandsson K, Drobnjak I, et al. Framework for the construction of a Monte Carlo simulated brain PET–MR image database. Nucl Instrum Methods Phys Res A 2014;734:162–5.

MR-Based Cardiac and Respiratory Motion-Compensation Techniques for PET-MR Imaging

Camila Munoz, MSc*, Christoph Kolbitsch, PhD,
Andrew J. Reader, PhD, Paul Marsden, PhD,
Tobias Schaeffter, PhD, Claudia Prieto, PhD

KEYWORDS

- Motion compensation • Respiratory motion • Cardiac motion • PET-MR imaging

KEY POINTS

- Recently developed simultaneous PET-MR scanners have broadened the possibilities for new MR-based motion-compensation techniques in PET.
- Two approaches have been proposed to use MR-measured motion fields to reconstruct a motion-corrected PET image: post-reconstruction registration and motion-compensated image reconstruction.
- MR-based motion-correction techniques for PET imaging improve the accuracy of uptake values and increase lesion detectability and contrast.
- Validation of the techniques in clinical studies with larger cohorts of patients remains to be done.

INTRODUCTION

Continuous improvement in clinical PET scanners has allowed attainment of an intrinsic spatial resolution in the range of 2 to 5 mm full-width-at-half-maximum (FWHM).[1] In practice, however, this resolution usually cannot be achieved when imaging the thoracic and abdominal regions, in part because of physiologic motion. Bulk patient motion during long PET acquisition times, as well as cardiac and respiratory motion, can have a negative effect on image quality and therefore diagnostic accuracy in a high number of patients. In addition to producing blurring, motion can produce severe image artifacts caused by mismatches between the static attenuation map and the moving emission map.[2] In oncology, motion affects ·the detectability of small lesions and the

accuracy of quantitative analysis, impairing diagnosis and therapy monitoring.[3,4] In cardiovascular imaging, severe attenuation map mismatches caused by motion may lead to the detection of false myocardial perfusion defects, as shown by Ouyang and colleagues[5] in **Fig. 1**.

Effects of cardiac motion are usually reduced in PET imaging by gating the acquisition into frames representing different cardiac phases. Typically, an external electrocardiogram (ECG) device is used to synchronize the acquisition with the cardiac cycle. The R-wave is used as a gating reference to estimate the cardiac phase in which each coincidence was acquired, thereby allowing the data to be sorted into near motion-free cardiac frames. This sorting can be performed retrospectively in scanners with list-mode acquisition capability, or prospectively (known as on-the-fly

Disclosure: The authors have nothing to disclose.
Division of Imaging Sciences and Biomedical Engineering, Department of Biomedical Engineering, King's College London, St. Thomas' Hospital, 4th Floor, Lambeth Wing, Westminster Bridge Road, London SE1 7EH, UK
* Corresponding author.
E-mail address: camila.munoz@kcl.ac.uk

PET Clin 11 (2016) 179–191
http://dx.doi.org/10.1016/j.cpet.2015.09.004
1556-8598/16/$ – see front matter

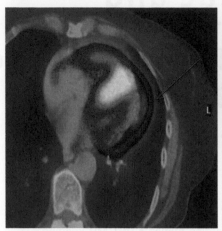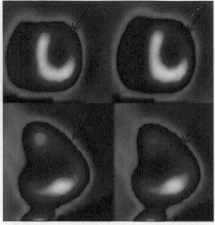

Fig. 1. Effect of motion in PET images. Arrows show an apparent myocardial perfusion defect. No stenosis was seen on subsequent catheterization or repeated imaging. (*From* Ouyang J, Li Q, El Fakhri G. Magnetic resonance-based motion correction for positron emission tomography imaging. Semin Nucl Med 2013;43:61; with permission.)

ECG-triggered acquisition). However, the signal-to-noise ratio (SNR) of each cardiac phase is highly reduced because of the low number of detected counts used in the individual reconstructions. An analogous approach can be used for respiratory motion compensation combining data acquired at similar respiratory positions from multiple breathing cycles. Usually, to measure the internal motion caused by the respiratory cycle directly is either not possible or difficult. Instead, data that can be easily measured (eg, the displacement of the skin surface) and that has a strong relationship with the motion of interest can be used as a respiratory surrogate.[6] As reviewed by Rahmim and colleagues,[1] different instrumentation solutions have been proposed to obtain a reliable surrogate signal that can be used for respiratory gating (also called binning). This includes pneumatic respiratory bellows, patient's airflow thermometers, infrared tracking systems that estimate the position of reflective markers placed in the patient's abdomen, or PET-based tracking systems where a radioactive point source is set on the patient's abdomen. Schemes that estimate a surrogate signal from PET data have also been proposed.[7] Most respiratory motion surrogates provide only qualitative information about different motion phases, which is not necessarily quantitatively linked to the motion of individual organs.

Cardiac and respiratory gating approaches have successfully been used in a wide range of static PET acquisitions,[1] where the reduced number of counts detected in each frame is compensated for by increasing acquisition time. However, this approach it is not suitable for four-dimensional (4D) dynamic PET studies. Temporal information about the radiopharmaceutical distribution is

sought in 4D dynamic PET, therefore acquisition time cannot be used as a resource to improve SNR. Furthermore, external devices do not measure internal motion directly and the information obtained from them is not directly suitable for motion-correction schemes.

Motion-correction techniques are required to overcome the SNR limitations of the gating approach. Some methods that estimate motion from PET data itself have been proposed.[8,9] However, such approaches have 2 main drawbacks: they assume that changes in the activity distribution are only caused by motion and their accuracy is limited by the inherent low spatial resolution of PET images which usually depends on the uptake of the radiotracer. In combined PET-computed tomography (CT) imaging, 4D CT has been proposed to estimate the motion and correct for it in the PET reconstruction.[10–13] Motion problems can be particularly challenging in PET-CT because images with the 2 modalities can only be obtained sequentially and not simultaneously, which can lead to spatial misalignment if not adequately addressed. Moreover, even if this problem can be solved, this approach significantly increases the total radiation dose to the patient.[10]

Recently developed whole-body PET-MR scanners have broadened the possibilities for new motion-compensation techniques in PET. MR imaging provides high-resolution images and superior soft-tissue contrast compared with CT, and can be acquired truly simultaneously with PET. Well-established techniques to estimate and compensate for motion in MR imaging can be applied to PET, without increasing radiation dose or total acquisition time.[14] Moreover, MR-measured motion fields can be used to correct both the PET emission data, to reduce image blurring and increase lesion detectability, and the attenuation maps to improve quantitative accuracy of the images.

This article reviews and discusses MR-based motion-compensation techniques that have been proposed to overcome the problem of cardiac and respiratory motion in PET-MR imaging. First, an overview of MR-based motion-estimation techniques that have been used for PET-MR is given. Then different techniques for motion correction of PET images in PET-MR are described. Preliminary results of the relative impact on image quality and quantitative accuracy of motion correction compared with other correction techniques are then presented. Finally, some areas of future work are discussed.

MR-BASED MOTION ESTIMATION

Motion measurements are challenging in the thoracic and abdominal regions because of nonrigid deformations of the organs during respiratory and cardiac cycles. Different approaches have been proposed to estimate cardiac and respiratory motion, ranging from simple one-dimensional (1D) signals that can be used for data binning to complex patient-specific models that provide 4D nonrigid motion information.

Most of the proposed techniques can be divided into 2 groups: (1) precalibrated motion model techniques that acquire dynamic MR data before or during the first minutes of the PET acquisition to form a patient-specific motion model and then acquire a surrogate during the PET acquisition; and (2) simultaneous motion model techniques, where motion is estimated using MR images that are acquired throughout the whole PET acquisition process.

Cardiac Motion

In the realm of MR imaging, the most widely used techniques to estimate cardiac motion are cine-MR imaging and tagged MR imaging.[15] In cine-MR imaging, data are acquired continuously throughout several cardiac cycles and are retrospectively binned into several motion-free cardiac phases using a simultaneously acquired ECG signal. Cine-MR imaging provides information for both motion estimation and functional assessment. In terms of motion estimation for PET-MR, cine-MR imaging can be classified as a simultaneous motion model technique. Two-dimensional (2D) fast low-angle shot (FLASH) cine-MR images have been used to estimate cardiac motion in a phantom PET-MR study, using B-spline nonrigid registration of 25 cardiac

phases with respect to an arbitrary reference phase.[16] Simulated three-dimensional (3D) T1-weighted images were also used by Tang and colleagues,[17] where an optical flow framework was used to estimate motion between 8 cardiac phases and the end-diastolic phase. The main drawback of the multiple 2D acquisition approach is that no information about 3D motion is available, so errors caused by misalignment between slices can be produced. Furthermore, motion is difficult to track in regions with uniform contrast such as the myocardium.

In tagged MR imaging, radiofrequency pre-pulses are used to generate a pattern of alternating bright and dark stripes. The most commonly used tagged MR imaging techniques are based on spatial modulation of magnetization (SPAMM), proposed by Axel and Dougherty,[18] where the deformation of a sinusoidal pattern superimposed on 2D images can be used to visualize and track motion. The pattern fades after the tagging prepulse as a result of relaxation processes, so multiple acquisitions are required in order to characterize the entire cardiac cycle. Furthermore, in order to track the 3D motion of the heart, multiple orthogonal image planes (ie, coronal, sagittal, transverse) or orthogonally motion-encoded volumes[19] need to be acquired. For this reason, tagged MR images are simultaneously acquired with an external ECG signal that allows for the triggering of the tagging prepulse and gating of the data in different cardiac phases, as can be seen in the schematic sequence in **Fig. 2**.

Once the tagged MR images have been reconstructed for each cardiac phase, different approaches can be used to estimate motion. B-spline nonrigid registration of SPAMM-tagged images has successfully been applied to track myocardial motion in PET-MR phantom studies,[5,20] and recently in a proof-of-concept clinical study[21] dividing the cardiac cycle into 9 phases.

One of the main disadvantages of tagged MR imaging is the extended time required to obtain a complete description of the motion during the cardiac cycle, so it is usually a simultaneous motion model technique. As reported,[21] the acquisition time of fully sampled tagged MR images for a patient experiment was more than 8 minutes, preventing the application of other clinically relevant sequences to assess cardiac anatomy and function. Half *k*-space acquisition,[20] compressed sensing, and parallel imaging undersampled reconstruction techniques[21] have been used to accelerate the acquisition of tagged MR images and move toward a precalibrated motion model approach. Huang and colleagues[21] demonstrated that using compressed sensing,[22] 8 times

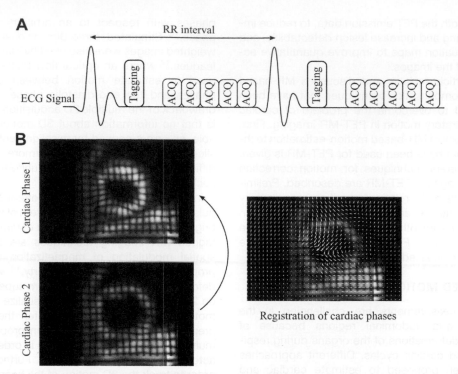

Fig. 2. (*A*) Schematic sequence of tagged MR imaging acquisition. (*B*) Two cardiac phases acquired using tagged MR images of a single ventricle patient are shown. Registration between cardiac phases provides an estimation of the motion fields.

accelerated tagged MR imaging can still provide accurate motion estimation and yield motion-corrected PET images of a similar quality to those corrected with motion estimated from fully sampled tagged MR imaging. This was demonstrated both in phantom studies and in 1 patient using myocardial defect contrast as the measurement of image quality. These preliminary results are promising; however, an increased sample size and standardized metrics of image quality for the motion-corrected PET image, such as channelized Hotelling observer (CHO),[23] are required in order to fully evaluate the performance of accelerated tagged MR imaging techniques.

Respiratory Motion

Breathing is the main source of motion in abdominal and thoracic imaging, and is a major problem in cardiac imaging. A wide variety of techniques have been proposed to estimate respiratory motion using MR images; however, this review focuses only on those that have been applied to PET-MR imaging.

As explained before, precalibrated motion model techniques aim to create a patient-specific motion model from imaging data, usually

by acquiring a surrogate signal simultaneously with the imaging data, so that the model approximates the relationship between the surrogate and the motion.[6] For PET-MR imaging, precalibrated motion models are based on near real-time MR images acquired before the simultaneous PET-MR acquisition. This approach has been applied in MR-based PET simulation studies[24–29] with healthy volunteer MR data. 3D T1-weighted turbo field echo (TFE) MR images were acquired using parallel imaging (SENSE) with an acceleration factor of 8, so that each whole-thorax volume is acquired in 0.7 seconds. Motion displacements estimated from hierarchical local affine registration of these fast acquired 3D MR imaging volumes are modeled as second-order polynomial functions of a 1D surrogate signal, so that during PET-MR acquisition only information from the position of a 1D navigator echo is required for motion estimation. In the report by King and colleagues,[30] 2D images were used as surrogate for a statistical motion model, and more robust results were obtained compared with 1D surrogates.

A different precalibrated model-based approach was proposed by Würslin and colleagues[31] and tested in thoracic images of 5 patients. Here, a motion model is generated during the first 3 minutes of simultaneous PET-MR acquisition, by acquiring multiple high-resolution 2D sagittal spoiled gradient echo MR images that are retrospectively reordered to form 4 3D volumes. During the remainder of the examination, only a 1D respiratory surrogate is acquired, which is used to retrospectively bin the acquired PET data. Motion fields are estimated by nonrigid registration of the 3D volumes to the end-expiratory volume. The investigators stated that reducing the time required for motion estimation was desirable in order to provide time for diagnostic MR sequences; however, there was no discussion about the effect of changing the time allocated for generating the motion model.

The most common simultaneous motion model approach applies nonrigid registration to images reconstructed at different respiratory bins (so-called bin-to-bin respiratory motion estimation). Similar to cardiac motion estimation, a signal related to the breathing cycle is required for retrospectively assigning the acquired data to different binning windows, so that each of the respiratory phases contains data acquired at similar respiratory positions in multiple breathing cycles. External devices can be used for this purpose, but MR imaging offers the capability of directly monitoring the hemidiaphragm position by interleaving 1D navigator echoes during MR acquisition. A navigator echo usually consists of an image of 1 thin column of tissue, obtained by applying a spatially selective excitation 2D pulse oriented in the foot-head direction, to monitor the position of the liver-lung interface. This approach has been used in 2 PET-MR patient studies. In the report by Dutta and colleagues,[32] data acquired using a golden-angle radial FLASH pulse sequence were retrospectively binned into 8 respiratory bins for thoracic imaging. In article by Petibon and colleagues,[33] data acquired using a navigated steady-state free-precession (true fast imaging with steady-state precession) MR acquisition protocol were binned into 7 bins for abdominal imaging.

Alternatively, a self-gating 1D respiratory surrogate to bin the data can be derived from the acquired data, without requiring additional interleaved echoes or external signals. A self-gating approach for respiratory motion estimation in PET-MR was proposed by Grimm and colleagues,[34,35] and evaluated in abdominal and thoracic images of 15 patients. MR data were acquired using a 3D T1-weighted golden-radial stack-of-stars spoiled gradient echo with fat suppression sequence. The stack-of-stars trajectory (Fig. 3) allows a respiratory signal to be derived from the center of the k-space ($k_x = k_y = 0$) for

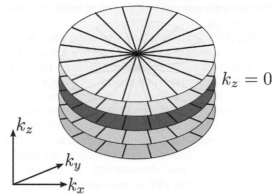

Fig. 3. The stacks-of-stars trajectory acquires radial spokes in the k_x–k_y plane and uses Cartesian sampling along the k_z direction. The angle increment between consecutively acquired spokes corresponds to the golden angle (111.246°). A respiratory signal can be estimated using the central sample of any spoke acquired in the central slice of the volume ($k_z = 0$).

each line acquired in the central slice of the volume ($k_z = 0$). Based on this signal the MR data were retrospectively binned into 2 to 15 uniform respiratory bins. The investigators concluded that up to 10 bins are required to recover the full respiratory amplitude depending on the respiratory pattern of the patient. However, when analyzing the average binning error, using only 5 bins the 95th percentile of the error was less than 2 mm, suggesting that increasing the number of bins to more than 5 does not have a significant impact on the accuracy of the estimated motion.

Fürst and colleagues[36] compared the performance of a simultaneous motion model using 5 different 1D respiratory surrogates for retrospective binning of MR data, including respiratory bellows, an MR-based self-gated signal, and 3 PET-based navigators, finding high correlation between the different respiratory signals. This study was performed in 20 patients, who were referred for diagnosis of malignant diseases in the abdomen (11 patients), heart (1 patient), and thorax (8 patients).

A different bin-to-bin-based simultaneous motion model approach involves the acquisition of near real-time MR images that are subsequently classified in different respiratory phases. Fieseler and colleagues,[16] used an image-based navigator to select 6 respiratory phases from a set of 35 acquired 3D TFE images of a phantom capable of both cardiac and respiratory motion. A similar approach was used by Manber and colleagues[37] for 2D motion estimation, where a PET-derived respiratory signal is used to group acquired 2D real-time MR images into 10 respiratory bins. Finally, motion is estimated by nonrigid registration between the average image of each bin and a reference image.

Tagged MR imaging has also been used to estimate respiratory motion to improve accuracy in regions with uniform contrast such as the liver. B-spline nonrigid registration of tagged MR images using 2 different similarity measures (ie, sum of squared differences and negative mutual information) has been applied to abdominal imaging of rabbits and nonhuman primates.[38] The investigators found no statistically significant difference in the detectability of lesions in motion-corrected PET images using either similarity measure. Guerin and colleagues[39] estimated motion through regularized phase-tracking of multislice tagged MR images. The proposed approach was demonstrated to be robust against noise in a numerical simulation study, but its applicability to in vivo data has not been tested. As discussed by the investigators, a severe limitation of tagged MR approaches for respiratory motion estimation is the lack of signal in the lungs.

Dual gating has been proposed to address both cardiac and respiratory motion simultaneously. Nonrigid registration of dual-gated images into a reference cardiac and respiratory phase, assuming the existence of 1D surrogates for both the cardiac-induced and respiratory-induced motion of the heart (**Fig. 4**), has been shown in simulation studies.[40,41] In the report by Tang and colleagues,[17] respiratory motion was assumed to be rigid within each cardiac phase, so rotation and translation parameters that characterize motion between respiratory phases were estimated using least squares minimization. Using these parameters, respiratory corrected MR images were reconstructed for each cardiac phase and, subsequently, nonrigid cardiac motion was estimated using optical flow.

Whereas simultaneous motion model techniques are robust for patients with irregular breathing patterns, they require continuous acquisition of motion information preventing the simultaneous acquisition of other diagnostic MR images during PET acquisition. However, precalibrated motion model techniques should allow the acquisition of different MR sequences in parallel with PET, when the required respiratory surrogate is 1D and can be obtained as part of the diagnostic MR acquisition. It is worth considering that although motion models provide near real-time motion estimates, motion correction is usually performed in a bin-to-bin framework because of computational constraints.

All previously described techniques assume that cardiac and respiratory motion is periodic, so that information about the relative position within the cardiac cycle and/or the respiratory cycle is enough to characterize the motion status of the acquired data. Nevertheless, during long examinations, images are also affected by bulk motion of the patient. The problem of detecting and

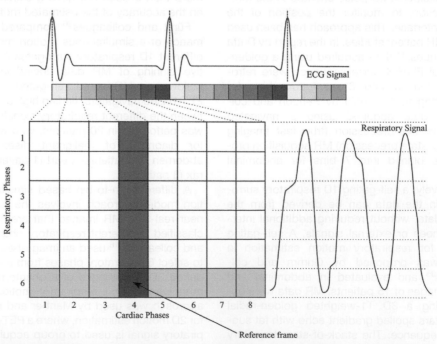

Fig. 4. Simultaneous cardiac and respiratory motion estimation from dual-gated MR data. Each motion-free frame is registered to a reference frame, usually end expiration and end-diastole.

estimating bulk motion in PET-MR has been addressed in a PET simulation study based on abdominal MR data from 3 healthy volunteers.[42] In vivo studies are required to assess the impact of bulk motion correction.

PET MOTION CORRECTION

MR-based estimated motion fields can be applied in 2 different ways to compensate for nonrigid motion in PET images. In the first, each motion-free frame is reconstructed independently, and inverse motion transformations are used to warp PET images from different motion states to a common reference position. This approach is variously known as postreconstruction registration (PRR), reconstruct-register-average, or reconstruct-transform-average.[43] The second approach incorporates the motion information directly into the system matrix of the iterative PET reconstruction algorithm, and is known as motion-compensated image reconstruction (MCIR).[44]

Postreconstruction Registration

In order to reconstruct each frame separately, PRR approaches apply binning to the acquired PET data with the same gating signal and bins used for motion estimation. Usually, each frame is reconstructed using the standard ordered-subsets expectation-maximization (OSEM) algorithm.[45] Attenuation correction maps for each bin are computed from a static reference map by applying the corresponding motion transformation. Once all frames have been reconstructed, they are transformed back to the reference frame, usually end expiration and end-diastole, and ultimately averaged (**Fig. 5**).

This approach has been applied in simulation studies with a numerical phantom[40] and PET simulations based on real MR data.[24,25,46,47] Studies reported improvements in accuracy of uptake values in lesions and regions of interest (ROIs),[24,25] increased contrast (72.17%) and SNR (63.8%) for manually defined ROIs,[47] and increased normalized cross-correlation[46] compared with uncorrected images. When applied to real PET-MR data from phantoms,[16,48] a significant reduction in image artifacts has been reported. Preliminary studies on patients[31,34] reported increased SNR (28.1%) and reduction in apparent lesion volume (11.8%–26.5%) compared with uncorrected images, but reduced contrast (−11.3%) compared with gated images. As discussed by Würslin and colleagues,[31] the loss of contrast is probably related to remnant intrabin motion that reduces the quality of the images reconstructed at each respiratory phase, and ultimately

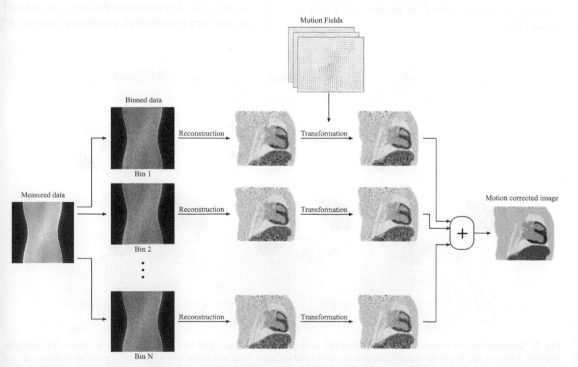

Fig. 5. Postreconstruction registration approach. The measured data are binned into *N* motion-free frames, which are reconstructed separately. Reconstructed images are then transformed to a reference frame using motion estimates, and finally averaged to obtain the final motion-corrected image.

induces blurring in the combined motion-corrected PET image (**Fig. 6**).

Instead of using the average of the back-transformed reconstructed frames, Grimm and colleagues[35] proposed the use of a weighted sum that takes into account the differences in image quality between frames. The weighting factor is inversely proportional to the intrabin amplitude range, so that quiescent respiratory gates such as end expiration have more influence in the final image than end-inspiratory data. However, results reported for lesions in 15 clinical patients still show reduced contrast (−10.3 ± 12.0%) compared with gated images (**Fig. 7**).

Motion-Corrected Image Reconstruction

Theoretically, once motion is available throughout the PET acquisition, PET data could be corrected by incorporating the transformation between the current and a reference position into any iterative reconstruction algorithm. However, in order to avoid increasing reconstruction time significantly, PET data are binned (**Fig. 8**). The widely used OSEM algorithm can be modified to include motion information in the system matrix, modifying both the emission and attenuation maps, as shown in Equation 1.[41] Accidental coincidences (ie, random and scatters) are usually assumed to vary slowly compared with the emission map, so the effect of motion on them is neglected.

$$\rho^{(iter+1)} = \frac{\rho^{(iter)}}{\sum_k (M^k)^T P^T NA^k 1_l}$$
$$\times \sum_k (M^k)^T P^T \frac{s_{tot}^k}{PM^k \rho^{(iter)} + (A^k N)^{-1} (\overline{sc} + \overline{r})} \quad (1)$$

where ρ is a column vector that contains the PET voxel values in the reference phase, M^k is a motion operator that transforms an image at the reference phase to a phase k, P is a matrix that models the system forward-projection, N is a diagonal matrix with entries down the diagonal equal to the reciprocal of the normalization-correction factors, A^k is a diagonal matrix with entries down the diagonal equal to the reciprocal of the attenuation correction factors for phase k, s_{tot}^k is a column vector that contains counts detected in phase k, and $\overline{sc}$, $\overline{r}$ represent estimations of scattered and random coincidences, respectively.

This approach has been applied in simulation studies with numerical phantoms,[28,49] PET simulation based on MR data of healthy volunteers,[41] PET-MR data acquired from phantoms,[20,39] animal studies,[5,38] and small studies on oncological and cardiac patients.[21,33,36,37] Phantom and animal studies reported that motion correction can improve contrast by 21% to 280% and lesion detectability by 19% to 235% compared with uncorrected images, and improves lesion detectability (65%–276%) compared with gated images. The wide range of improvement is probably related to the wide range of motion amplitudes studied. In

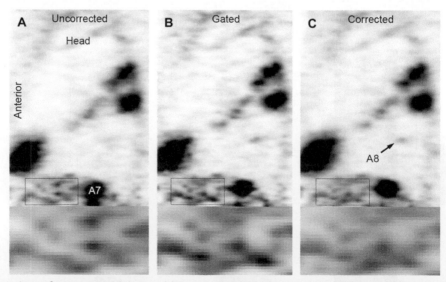

Fig. 6. Comparison of uncorrected (*A*), gated (*B*), and corrected (*C*) sagittal PET image slice of a lung with multiple lesions. Lesion (A8) is enhanced in gated and corrected images. Box indicates the zoomed region at bottom of the Figure. (This research was originally published in *JNM*. Würslin C, Schmidt H, Martirosian P, et al. Respiratory motion correction in oncologic PET using T1-weighted MR imaging on a simultaneous whole-body PET/MR system. J Nucl Med 2013;54(3):464–7. © by the Society of Nuclear Medicine and Molecular Imaging, Inc.)

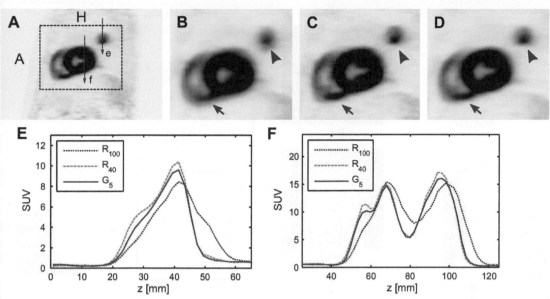

Fig. 7. (A) Sagittal slice through heart, (B) uncorrected image (R100), (C) gated image (R40), (D) motion-corrected image (G5). Motion correction reduces blurring compared with uncorrected reconstruction, but the contrast is not fully recovered as can be seen in the profiles through (E) the lesion (*arrowhead*) and (F) the myocardium (*arrow*). (*From* Grimm R, Fürst S, Souvatzoglou M, et al. Self-gated MRI motion modeling for respiratory motion compensation in integrated PET/MRI. Med Image Anal 2014;19:117; with permission.)

regions where motion is large, motion correction could have more impact than in regions with small or no motion. For patients, the results reported show an increase in the lesion uptake value of 11% to 23%, a reduction in the apparent lesion volume of 12% to 29%, and an increase in the SNR of 21% to 44% in comparison with uncorrected images. An example of the impact of motion correction in liver lesion detection can be seen in **Fig. 9.**[20] Improvements in contrast without SNR loss are apparent in the motion-corrected image. Besides motion-compensated OSEM, iterative motion-compensated maximum a posteriori (MAP) image reconstruction has also been proposed.[32]

Tang and colleagues[17] used a combination of PRR and MCIR approaches. For a dual-gated simulated PET-MR dataset, each cardiac phase was reconstructed using respiratory motion-compensated OSEM, and then cardiac phases were transformed and averaged to obtain the final image. The investigators found improved lesion detectability for motion-corrected images compared with uncorrected data (12.9%), and for each respiratory corrected cardiac gate compared with dual-gated images (21.4%).

Comparison Between Motion-Compensated Image Reconstruction and Postreconstruction Registration

To summarize, all studies reviewed report that MR-based cardiac and respiratory motion-

correction techniques reduce image blurring and improve contrast recovery compared with non–motion-corrected reconstruction, and improve SNR, and lesion detectability compared with gated reconstruction.

Of the available literature, approximately half used MCIR. Only simulation studies have compared the performance of both approaches. In a preliminary study by Dikaios and Fryer[50] based on pseudo-PET images generated from real abdominal and thoracic MR data, less bias in organ uptake values was obtained using MCIR. Using PET simulations based on MR data of 2 volunteers in a more recent study,[51] they concluded that PRR produces greater resolution loss than MCIR, but they have comparable performance in terms of global similarity indices (root mean squared error, correlation coefficient, and normalized mutual information) with respect to a motion-free gold standard.

Polycarpou and colleagues[26,27] and Tsoumpas and colleagues[29] also performed a comparison between the 2 approaches using OSEM reconstruction in an MR-based PET simulation study. They found that MCIR achieves better contrast and smaller bias in low-activity regions compared with PRR, but has lower SNR. For a small number of iterations (ie, 1–2), MCIR has better performance in terms of mean squared error (MSE) than PRR. However, as the number of iterations increases, PRR has significantly less MSE than

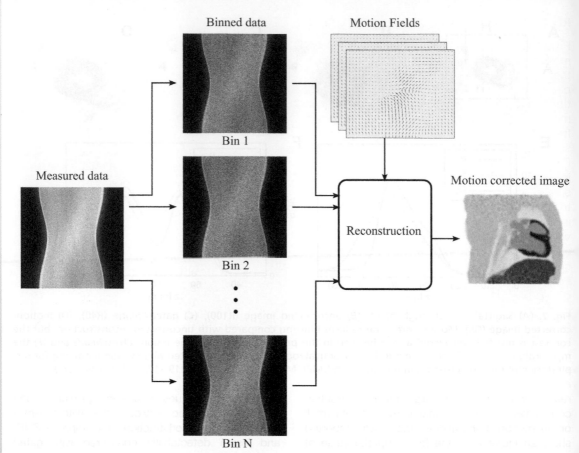

Fig. 8. Motion-compensated image reconstruction approach. The iterative reconstruction algorithm is modified in order to include motion information, modifying both the emission and attenuation maps. Usually, data are binned into motion-free frames to reduce computational burden of the reconstruction.

MCIR. This suggests that in cases where SNR is high, MCIR may provide better performance. Alternatively, regularization methods can be incorporated in PET reconstruction to control noise levels. As shown in an MR-based PET simulation study,[52] when using the ordered-subsets MAP 1-step-late algorithm with median-root-prior, MCIR with optimized regularization parameters achieves less bias and MSE, and similar contrast and SNR compared with regularized PRR.

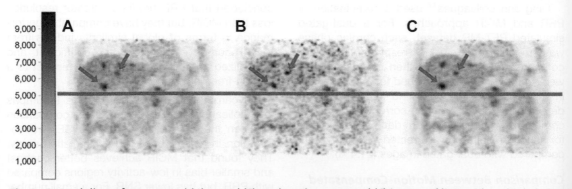

Fig. 9. Coronal slices of uncorrected (*A*), gated (*B*), and motion-corrected (*C*) images of liver with multiple lesions (*arrows*). Motion blurring of lesions was significantly reduced by gating and motion correction; however, increased noise in the gated image reduces lesion detectability. (This research was originally published in *JNM*. Fürst S, Grimm R, Hong I, et al. Motion correction strategies for integrated PET/MR. J Nucl Med 2015;56(2):261–9. © by the Society of Nuclear Medicine and Molecular Imaging, Inc.)

RELATIVE IMPACT OF MOTION CORRECTION

Preliminary studies to assess the relative impact of motion correction compared with other factors that affect the quality of PET images have been performed. Buerger and colleagues[24] compared the impact of motion and errors in the attenuation map in a PET simulation study using real MR data from 5 healthy volunteers, finding that both have a similar effect on standardized uptake values. Petibon and colleagues[33] studied the impact of including a spatially dependent model of the point spread function (PSF) into the reconstruction, testing 4 reconstruction algorithms in abdominal images of 3 patients: standard OSEM, OSEM with PSF modeling, motion-corrected OSEM, and OSEM with both PSF modeling and motion correction. The investigators concluded that the enhancement offered by PSF modeling in terms of FWHM and SNR is more significant when correcting for motion at the same time. Finally, Polycarpou and colleagues[28,49] simulated different scanner resolutions (3 and 6 mm), finding that the benefit of having higher scanner resolution is small unless motion-correction techniques are applied.

AREAS OF FUTURE RESEARCH

MR-based motion correction for PET-MR imaging is an emerging field of research, and several questions about performance and the impact of proposed approaches still remain unanswered. Most of the revised techniques have been validated in simulations, ad hoc phantoms, or small patient cohorts. Studies with standardized thoracic and abdominal phantoms capable of cardiac and/or respiratory motion are required to validate motion-estimation techniques and the accuracy of motion-corrected images.

Different clinical applications of PET have different image quality requirements. For example, lesion detectability and accurate uptake values are relevant in oncological applications, whereas improved spatial resolution is essential for some cardiovascular applications such as coronary artery imaging. For this reason, application-specific studies with larger sample sizes are required to evaluate the impact of motion correction.

Another issue that needs to be addressed is the optimal number of respiratory and cardiac phases. Reported techniques have used 4 to 8 respiratory bins and 8 to 25 cardiac gates. Grimm and colleagues[34,35] studied the average binning error for different numbers of respiratory bins; however, the impact on the motion-corrected PET image was not addressed.

In most studies, motion fields are estimated only from MR data. Motion fields estimated from both PET and MR data have been used in a simulation study,[40] showing local improvements in motion-estimation accuracy near lesions and other regions with significant tracer uptake. The impact of this technique in real PET-MR data remains to be studied.

Finally, state-of-the-art literature in PET-MR motion correction only uses MR data for motion-estimation purposes. In most cases, motion fields estimated from MR have been used to correct PET data, but no correction is performed in the simultaneously acquired MR data. Kolbitsch and colleagues[42] reported a scheme for bulk motion compensation of both PET and MR images; however, this approach has not been applied to cardiac or respiratory motion. A different approach has been proposed,[53] whereby motion is jointly estimated during MR image reconstruction, and subsequently applied to correct simulated PET data. Furthermore, design of MR protocols and techniques that make the acquisition of information useful for both motion estimation and diagnosis is still an open area.

SUMMARY

In this article, techniques that estimate cardiac and respiratory motion from MR data to perform motion correction of PET images in the context of cardiac, thoracic, and abdominal PET-MR imaging have been reviewed.

Different techniques have been proposed to obtain estimates of cardiac and respiratory motion. For abdominal and thoracic imaging, pre-calibrated motion models and simultaneously acquired motion models are the most common approaches for respiratory motion estimation. For cardiac imaging, some approaches only address cardiac motion through nonrigid registration of tagged or cine-MR images gated with an external ECG device. In order to include respiratory motion of the heart, nonrigid registration of dual-gated MR images has been used.

Once an estimate of the motion is available, 2 approaches to correct PET data have been proposed. In PRR, each motion-free frame is reconstructed independently, and images are then combined using motion estimates. However, in MCIR, the motion information is directly incorporated into the system matrix directly reconstructing a motion-corrected image. Using either of them significantly increases lesion detectability and contrast without SNR loss. In addition, improved accuracy of uptake values has been reported for simulation, phantom, and preclinical as well as preliminary patient studies.

REFERENCES

1. Rahmim A, Rousset O, Zaidi H. Strategies for motion tracking and correction in PET. PET Clin 2007;2(2):251–66.

2. Papathanassiou D, Becker S, Amir R, et al. Respiratory motion artefact in the liver dome on FDG PET/CT: comparison of attenuation correction with CT and a caesium external source. Eur J Nucl Med Mol Imaging 2005;32(12):1422–8.

3. Liu C, Pierce LA, Alessio AM, et al. The impact of respiratory motion on tumor quantification and delineation in static PET/CT imaging. Phys Med Biol 2009;54(24):7345–62.

4. Nehmeh SA, Erdi YE, Ling CC, et al. Effect of respiratory gating on quantifying PET images of lung cancer. J Nucl Med 2002;43(7):876–81.

5. Ouyang J, Li Q, El Fakhri G. Magnetic resonance-based motion correction for positron emission tomography imaging. Semin Nucl Med 2013;43(1):60–7.

6. McClelland JR, Hawkes DJ, Schaeffter T, et al. Respiratory motion models: a review. Med Image Anal 2013;17(1):19–42.

7. Schleyer PJ, O'Doherty MJ, Barrington SF, et al. Retrospective data-driven respiratory gating for PET/CT. Phys Med Biol 2009;54(7):1935–50.

8. Klein GJ, Reutter BW, Huesman RH. Four-dimensional affine registration models for respiratory-gated PET. IEEE Trans Nucl Sci 2001;48(3):756–60.

9. Ambwani S, Karl WC, Tawakol A, et al. Joint cardiac and respiratory motion correction and super-resolution reconstruction in coronary PET/CT. Presented at the 2011 IEEE International Symposium on Biomedical Imaging: From Nano to Macro. Chicago, IL, March 30 – April 2, 2011. p. 1702–5.

10. Nehmeh SA, Erdi YE. Respiratory motion in positron emission tomography/computed tomography: a review. Semin Nucl Med 2008;38(3):167–76.

11. McQuaid SJ, Lambrou T, Cunningham VJ, et al. The application of a statistical shape model to diaphragm tracking in respiratory-gated cardiac pet images. Proc IEEE 2009;97(12):2039–52.

12. McQuaid SJ, Lambrou T, Hutton BF. A novel method for incorporating respiratory-matched attenuation correction in the motion correction of cardiac PET-CT studies. Phys Med Biol 2011;56(10):2903–15.

13. Fayad HJ, Pan T, Roux C, et al. A generic respiratory motion model for motion correction in PET/CT. Presented at the IEEE Nuclear Science Symposuim & Medical Imaging Conference. Knoxville, TN, October 30 – November 6, 2010. p. 2455–8.

14. Quick HH. Integrated PET/MR. J Magn Reson Imaging 2014;39(2013):243–58.

15. Wang H, Amini AA. Cardiac motion and deformation recovery from MRI: a review. IEEE Trans Med Imaging 2012;31(2):487–503.

16. Fieseler M, Kugel H, Gigengack F, et al. A dynamic thorax phantom for the assessment of cardiac and respiratory motion correction in PET/MRI: a preliminary evaluation. Nucl Instrum Methods Phys Res A 2012;702:59–63.

17. Tang J, Hall N, Rahmim A. MRI assisted motion correction in dual-gated 5D myocardial perfusion PET imaging. Presented at the 2012 IEEE Nuclear Science Symposium and Medical Imaging Conference Record (NSS/MIC). Anaheim, CA, October 27 – November 3, 2012. p. 4054–7.

18. Axel L, Dougherty L. MR imaging of motion with spatial modulation of magnetization. Radiology 1989;171(3):841–5.

19. Rutz AK, Ryf S, Plein S, et al. Accelerated whole-heart 3D CSPAMM for myocardial motion quantification. Magn Reson Med 2008;59(4):755–63.

20. Petibon Y, Ouyang J, Zhu X, et al. Cardiac motion compensation and resolution modeling in simultaneous PET-MR: a cardiac lesion detection study. Phys Med Biol 2013;58(7):2085–102.

21. Huang C, Petibon Y, Ouyang J, et al. Accelerated acquisition of tagged MRI for cardiac motion correction in simultaneous PET-MR: phantom and patient studies. Med Phys 2015;42(2):1087–97.

22. Lustig M, Donoho D, Pauly JM. Sparse MRI: the application of compressed sensing for rapid MR imaging. Magn Reson Med 2007;58(6):1182–95.

23. Barrett HH, Yao J, Rolland JP, et al. Model observers for assessment of image quality. Proc Natl Acad Sci U S A 1993;90(21):9758–65.

24. Buerger C, Tsoumpas C, Aitken A, et al. Investigation of MR-based attenuation correction and motion compensation for hybrid PET/MR. IEEE Trans Nucl Sci 2012;59(5):1967–76.

25. King AP, Tsoumpas C, Buerger C, et al. Real-time respiratory motion correction for simultaneous PET-MR using an MR-derived motion model. Presented at the 2011 IEEE Nuclear Science Symposium and Medical Imaging Conference. Valencia, October 23–29, 2011. p. 3589–94.

26. Polycarpou I, Tsoumpas C, Marsden PK. Analysis and comparison of two methods for motion correction in PET imaging. Med Phys 2012;39(10):6474–83.

27. Polycarpou I, Tsoumpas C, Marsden PK. Statistical evaluation of PET motion correction methods using MR derived motion fields. In IEEE Nuclear Science Symposium Conference. Valencia, October 23–29, 2011. p. 3579–85.

28. Polycarpou I, Tsoumpas C, King AP, et al. Impact of respiratory motion correction and spatial resolution on lesion detection in PET: a simulation study based on real MR dynamic data. Phys Med Biol 2014;59(3):697–713.

29. Tsoumpas C, Agarwal S, Marsden PK, et al. Evaluation of two PET motion correction techniques for simultaneous real-time PET-MR acquisitions using an MR-derived motion model. Presented at the IEEE Nuclear Science Symposium Conference. Anaheim, CA, October 27 – November 3, 2012. p. 2519–22.

30. King AP, Buerger C, Tsoumpas C, et al. Thoracic respiratory motion estimation from MRI using a statistical model and a 2-D image navigator. Med Image Anal 2012;16(1):252–64.

31. Würslin C, Schmidt H, Martirosian P, et al. Respiratory motion correction in oncologic PET using T1-weighted MR imaging on a simultaneous whole-body PET/MR system. J Nucl Med 2013;54(3):464–71.

32. Dutta J, El Fakhri G, Huang C, et al. Respiratory motion compensation in simultaneous PET/MR using a maximum a posteriori approach. Presented at the 2013 IEEE 10th International Symposium on Biomedical Imaging. San Francisco, CA, April 7–11, 2013. p. 800–3.

33. Petibon Y, Huang C, Ouyang J, et al. Relative role of motion and PSF compensation in whole-body oncologic PET-MR imaging. Med Phys 2014;41(4): 042503.

34. Grimm R, Fürst S, Dregely I, et al. Self-gated radial MRI for respiratory motion compensation on hybrid PET/MR systems. In: Mori K, Sakuma I, Sato Y, et al, editors. Medical image computing and computer-assisted intervention – MICCAI 2013 SE - 3, vol. 8151. Berlin; Heidelberg (Germany): Springer; 2013. p. 17–24.

35. Grimm R, Fürst S, Souvatzoglou M, et al. Self-gated MRI motion modeling for respiratory motion compensation in integrated PET/MRI. Med Image Anal 2014;19(1):110–20.

36. Fürst S, Grimm R, Hong I, et al. Motion correction strategies for integrated PET/MR. J Nucl Med 2015;56:261–9.

37. Manber R, Thielemans K, Hutton BF, et al. Initial evaluation of a practical PET respiratory motion correction method in clinical simultaneous PET/MRI. EJNMMI Phys 2014;1(Suppl 1):A40.

38. Chun SY, Reese TG, Ouyang J, et al. MRI-based nonrigid motion correction in simultaneous PET/MRI. J Nucl Med 2012;53(8):1284–91.

39. Guerin B, Cho S, Chun SY, et al. Nonrigid PET motion compensation in the lower abdomen using simultaneous tagged-MRI and PET imaging. Med Phys 2011;38(6):3025–38.

40. Fieseler M, Gigengack F, Jiang X, et al. Motion correction of whole-body PET data with a joint PET-MRI registration functional. Biomed Eng Online 2014;13(Suppl 1):S2.

41. Petibon Y, El Fakhri G, Nezafat R, et al. Towards coronary plaque imaging using simultaneous PET-MR: a simulation study. Phys Med Biol 2014; 59(5):1203–22.

42. Kolbitsch C, Prieto C, Tsoumpas C, et al. A 3D MR-acquisition scheme for nonrigid bulk motion correction in simultaneous PET-MR. Med Phys 2014;41(8): 082304.

43. Picard Y, Thompson CJ. Motion correction of PET images using multiple acquisition frames. IEEE Trans Med Imaging 1997;16(2):137–44.

44. Qiao F, Pan T, Clark JW, et al. A motion-incorporated reconstruction method for gated PET studies. Phys Med Biol 2006;51(15):3769–83.

45. Hudson HM, Larkin RS. Accelerated image reconstruction using ordered subsets of projection data. IEEE Trans Med Imaging 1994;13(4):601–9.

46. Miao S, Liao R, Moran G, et al. Dynamic MR-based respiratory motion compensation for hybrid PET/MR system. Presented at the 9th IEEE Conference on Industrial Electronics and Applications. Hangzhou, June 9–11, 2014. p. 1915–20.

47. Fayad HJ, Odille F, Felblinger J, et al. A generic PET/MRI respiratory motion correction using a generalized reconstruction by inversion of coupled systems (GRICS) approach. Presented at the 2012 IEEE Nuclear Science Symposium and Medical Imaging Conference Record (NSS/MIC). Anaheim, CA, October 27 – November 3, 2012. p. 2813–6.

48. Tsoumpas C, Mackewn JE, Halsted P, et al. Simultaneous PET-MR acquisition and MR-derived motion fields for correction of non-rigid motion in PET. Ann Nucl Med 2010;24(10):745–50.

49. Polycarpou I, Tsoumpas C, King AP, et al. Quantitative evaluation of PET respiratory motion correction using real- time PET/MR simulated data. EJNMMI Phys 2014;1(Suppl 1):A62.

50. Dikaios N, Fryer TD. Respiratory motion correction of PET using motion parameters from MR. Presented at the 2009 IEEE Nuclear Science Symposium Conference Record (NSS/MIC). Orlando, FL, October 24 – November 1, 2009. p. 2806–8.

51. Dikaios N, Izquierdo-Garcia D, Graves MJ, et al. MRI-based motion correction of thoracic PET: initial comparison of acquisition protocols and correction strategies suitable for simultaneous PET/MRI systems. Eur Radiol 2012;22(2):439–46.

52. Tsoumpas C, Polycarpou I, Thielemans K, et al. The effect of regularization in motion compensated PET image reconstruction: a realistic numerical 4D simulation study. Phys Med Biol 2013;58(6):1759–73.

53. Fayad HJ, Odille F, Schmidt H, et al. The use of a generalized reconstruction by inversion of coupled systems (GRICS) approach for generic respiratory motion correction in PET/MR imaging. Phys Med Biol 2015;60(6):2529–46.

MRI-Guided Derivation of the Input Function for PET Kinetic Modeling

Marie Anne Richard, BSc[a], Jérémie P. Fouquet, BSc[a],
Réjean Lebel, PhD[b], Martin Lepage, PhD[c,*]

KEYWORDS

- PET • MRI • Kinetic modeling • Image-derived input function • Input function conversion
- Arterial input function

KEY POINTS

- MRI can be used to segment PET images and correct partial volume effects to improve the image-derived input function.
- For simultaneous PET–MRI scans, the image-derived input function can be improved by MRI-guided motion correction.
- Preclinical studies have shown that the input function of Gd-DTPA can be converted into an fluo-rodeoxyglucose and a [18F]fluoroethyl-L-tyrosine input function.

INTRODUCTION

Knowledge of the arterial input function (AIF), that is, the concentration of a tracer in arterial blood over time, is a prerequisite of most pharmacokinetic models used in quantitative PET. However, the gold standard for AIF determination is arterial blood sampling, a complex, time-consuming, and invasive procedure that is not feasible in all subjects. Also, it is noteworthy that arterial sampling is rarely performed in an artery directly feeding the region of interest (ROI); therefore, the measured AIF may have to be adjusted for delay and dispersion. To circumvent these problems, the AIF can be derived from dynamic images using methods that involve no, or minimal, blood sampling.[1] All of these methods require precise knowledge of the tracer concentration in a specific region, making them dependent on image segmentation, partial volume effect (PVE) correction, and motion correction.

MRI is used frequently to perform segmentation, partial volume correction, and motion correction of coregistered PET images because it can provide high-resolution anatomic and perfusion images. It can also serve to identify major blood vessel on PET images[2] from which to extract the AIF. Moreover, preliminary studies indicate that an MRI contrast agent AIF could be used to calculate the PET tracer AIF[3,4] by applying simple conversion factors. Finally, with the emergence of simultaneous PET–MRI systems, spatial and temporal

Disclosure Statement: The authors have nothing to disclose.
[a] Department of Nuclear Medicine and Radiobiology, Centre d'imagerie moléculaire de Sherbrooke (CIMS), Université de Sherbrooke, Suite 1983, 3001, 12th Avenue North, Sherbrooke, Québec J1H 5N4, Canada;
[b] Department of Nuclear Medicine and Radiobiology, Centre d'imagerie moléculaire de Sherbrooke (CIMS), Université de Sherbrooke, Suite 1982, 3001, 12th Avenue North, Sherbrooke, Québec J1H 5N4, Canada;
[c] Department of Nuclear Medicine and Radiobiology, Centre d'imagerie moléculaire de Sherbrooke (CIMS), Université de Sherbrooke, 3001, 12th Avenue North, Sherbrooke, Québec J1H 5N4, Canada
* Corresponding author.
E-mail address: martin.lepage@usherbrooke.ca

PET Clin 11 (2016) 193–202
http://dx.doi.org/10.1016/j.cpet.2015.09.003
1556-8598/16/$ – see front matter © 2016 Elsevier Inc. All rights reserved.

registration of MR and PET images will become easier,[5] increasing the appeal of MRI-guided AIF extraction methods in the clinical setting.

This article provides a review of state-of-the art developments and techniques facilitating noninvasive PET kinetic modeling based on the image-derived AIF (IDAIF) in human subjects, either with sequential or simultaneous PET–MRI. The alternative method of PET–MRI AIF conversion is also discussed. Finally, limitations and advantages of the IDAIF for quantitative modeling are presented.

METHODOLOGY

The present article provides an overview of MRI-guided methods used to determine the PET IDAIF in humans, with an emphasis on the most recent developments. For this purpose, an exhaustive review of papers found on PubMed pertaining to clinical studies and corresponding to selected keywords (**Table 1**) was performed. It was also deemed appropriate to extend its scope and include articles on MRI-based segmentation and image correction methods for PET that could improve IDAIF determination. Findings from simulations and preclinical studies were added as complementary data. For the topic of AIF conversion, an exhaustive review of preclinical and clinical data was performed.

MRI-BASED SEGMENTATION

All IDAIF extraction methods are based on carefully selected ROIs. The ROI can be placed in a large blood pool or blood vessel[1,6] or in a region of reference (RR) showing no, or very little, specific interaction and a degree of nonspecific interaction similar to that of the ROI.[7] Delineation of the ROI must be precise to avoid signal contamination from surrounding tissues and to prepare further processing steps, such as PVE correction,[8] which

are discussed elsewhere in this article. Although it is possible to segment PET images directly, issues such as insufficient spatial resolution or lack of anatomic landmarks make the use of registered anatomic MR images more appealing.[9] Segmenting PET data based on MR images requires registering the PET and MR images and choosing the appropriate segmentation method for the type of RR and pulse sequence.

Registration

MRI-based PET segmentation methods rely on proper registration of images from both modalities. Small registration errors affect the IDAIF, and propagate to the quantitative measures (eg, rate constants, distribution volumes, binding potential, blood flow). For example, a registration error of 1° for the carotid arteries has been shown to affect the cerebral blood flow estimation based on the [^{15}O]-water IDAIF by approximately 10%.[2] Registration and segmentation errors are additive: simulations indicated that a total error of 2 MRI pixels (1.88 mm) between the simulated PET image and the corresponding 3D anatomic MR image may result in a deviation up to 15% from the expected gray matter tracer concentration.[10] The algorithms available for automatic registration[11] perform well for rigid brain registration with errors inferior to 2 mm and 1°.[12] Problems arise, however, when nonrigid deformations occur between the PET and MRI scans. For example, a slight head movement causes the carotid arteries to shift and deform in a way that cannot be corrected simply by registering brain images: independent registration of each artery must, therefore, be performed after brain registration.[13] In the case of a cardiac RR, the problem is even more complex because images have to be registered both in the spatial and the time domain.[14] Combined PET–MRI systems enabling simultaneous imaging

Table 1
Keywords used to filter the articles presented in this review

Key Concepts	Arterial Input Function	Image Derived	Kinetic Modeling	PET	MRI
Synonyms	Input function	Imaging-guided	Pharmacokinetic	PET	MRI
Abbreviation	AIF	Reference region	modeling (or modeling)		
Near-synonyms		RR	PKM		
		MRI-guided	PK		
		Reference tissue	Quantitative procedures		
			Quantification		

Abbreviations: AIF, arterial input function; PK, pharmacokinetic; PKM, pharmacokinetic modeling; RR, region of reference.

circumvent this issue for most pulse sequences, with the exception of sequences prone to image deformation, such as echoplanar imaging (EPI).[15,16]

Segmentation Methods

Image segmentation is a key step in the determination of IDAIFs. Segmentation can be achieved manually, semiautomatically, or automatically, the semiautomatic and automatic methods being preferred because they prove more reproducible and less time consuming for operators.[17] A complete review of these methods is beyond the scope of this article and interested readers will find relevant information in many excellent publications including those by Gordillo and colleagues,[17] Bauer and colleagues,[18] and Cabezas and colleagues.[19]

The choice of a segmentation method is based on some key aspects such as the type of RR, the type of image (eg, functional vs anatomic), and the subject population. Most often, MR images are segmented based on voxel similarity criteria or on atlases. On anatomic images, similarity criteria include notably signal intensity[2] or region smoothness.[9,13] To be effective, these methods require sufficient contrast between the RR and neighboring tissues. Similarity criteria based on signal enhancement over time after the injection of a contrast agent can also be used to segment arteries or an RR.[20–22] For neurologic applications, registration to an atlas allows finer segmentation of numerous anatomic and functional regions, provided that the atlas is representative of the population studied.[19] Moreover, a representative MRI atlas can be a stepping stone in the creation of a tracer-specific PET atlas[23] for direct PET image segmentation. Note that, depending on the segmentation method, the MRI pulse sequence must be optimized to provide adequate spatial resolution, temporal resolution, and/or contrast. For example, MR angiography, with its high contrast and spatial resolution, is particularly useful to delineate carotid or other major arteries (**Fig. 1**).[24]

MRI-BASED PARTIAL VOLUME CORRECTION

PVE can lead to errors in the estimation of an IDAIF. Currently, whole body clinical PET scanners can reach a spatial resolution of 4 to 5 mm full width at half maximum (FWHM),[25] whereas preclinical scanners approach 1 mm FWHM.[26] The theoretic limits, based solely on minimal positron range and acollinearity, are estimated at 1.83 and 0.67 mm FWHM, respectively, for clinical and preclinical scanners.[27] To avoid PVE, the object must be 2 to 3 times larger than the FWHM resolution of the scanner,[28] which is the case for larger heart vessels or ventricles in humans, but not for the carotid arteries (around 4–6 mm in diameter)[29] or for applications in small animals. Failure to correct for PVE induces errors in RR tracer concentration through signal contamination because several tissues can contribute to the signal of a voxel. For example, even if a tracer is purely intravascular, the signal seems to "leak" into neighboring tissues (an effect called spill-out), reducing the magnitude of the IDAIF. Inversely, if the concentration is higher in the surrounding tissues than in the arteries, the blood concentration seems higher than it really is (spill-in). Both the magnitude and shape of the IDAIF are modified by these effects. Errors on the rate constants without PVE correction are estimated to approximately 50% for a standard dynamic sequence acquired on a scanner with a 6-mm FWHM resolution followed by image reconstruction using filtered back projection.[30] The sub-millimeter in-plane resolution and soft tissue contrast of MRI can help to mitigate PVE by providing a priori anatomic information to mathematical models describing the contribution of each tissue type to the signal (**Fig. 2**). Different models exist for PVE correction depending on the anatomic features of interest (eg, vasculature or brain regions). To correct for PVE in the carotid artery, MR angiography and black-blood images can be used to evaluate the actual intravascular volume and position of the artery. These data, in combination with registered PET images and the point spread function of the scanner will provide an estimation of the PVE and allow the correction of the time–activity curve both for spill-in and spill-out.[24]

Whereas classic pharmacokinetic models assume that each voxel comprises a single tissue type and its feeding blood vessels, this is not always the case. For example, signals from white matter, gray matter, and cerebrospinal fluid must be separated. It then becomes critical to assess the contribution of each tissue type to the overall signal. To tackle this problem, Videen and colleagues[31] as well as Meltzer and colleagues[32] introduced a model, which was later refined by Müller-Gärtner and colleagues.[10] In this model, the observed radioactivity distribution is the convolution of the actual distribution and the point spread function of the scanner. In addition, radioactivity is considered to be uniform in each tissue type and is recovered from ROIs that are assumed to be devoid of PVE. The original radioactivity map is then obtained through deconvolution. However, the deconvolution process becomes impractical when considering a large number of heterogeneous

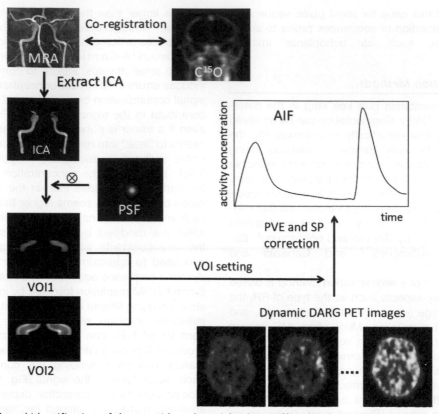

Fig. 1. MRI-based identification of the carotids and partial volume effect (PVE) correction in the semiautomated PET arterial input function extraction process presented by Iguchi and colleagues (2012) PET and MRI scans were conducted separately, increasing the importance of the registration step. DARG, dual-tracer autoradiographic method; PSF, point spread function; VOI, voxel of interest. (*From* Iguchi S, Hori Y, Moriguchi T, et al. Verification of a semi-automated MRI-guided technique for non-invasive determination of the arterial input function in ^{15}O-labeled gaseous PET. Nucl Instrum Methods Phys Res A 2013;702:112; with permission.)

tissue types (eg, when distinguishing between nonhomogeneous gray matter regions). Rousset and colleagues[33] provided an effective solution to account for the interaction of multiple tissues using a geometric transfer matrix method. An alternative to this method is the multiresolution approach where details from a high resolution anatomic image (MRI or computed tomography) are incorporated in the low resolution functional PET image through wavelet decomposition.[34–37] The 3D local multiresolution algorithm has proved as effective as the geometric transfer matrix method and does not require image segmentation.[36,37] However, accurate registration of both images and characterization of the point spread function are required for all of these methods.

MRI–BASED PET MOTION CORRECTION

The spatial accuracy and precision of PET and MR images is limited by motion. Consequently, cardiac and respiratory motion must be taken into account when selecting an RR in heart ventricles or large abdominal vessels. The same is true for head motion in brain imaging, where physical restraints cannot completely eliminate movement (eg, artery pulsation and residual patient movement). Motion induces blurring and complicates the previous steps of segmentation and PVE correction. It has been shown that the error on the IDAIF is important even in the case of small movement. For example, a 4-mm translation leads to about an 8% error on the distribution volume.[38] Also note that, in human subjects, both the PET image and the attenuation map must be corrected for motion.

To correct for motion in PET, conventional strategies include cardiac and respiratory gating[39] and head motion tracking using external sensors.[40] The main drawback of gating is increased noise owing to the limited duration of each gated frame. As for external sensors, they require precise positioning and a tracking device, such as a camera or the MRI itself in the case of combined PET–MRI

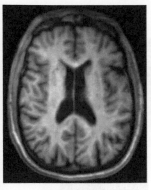
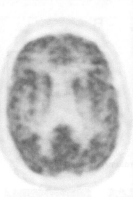
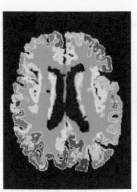
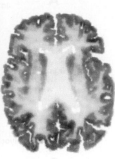

| Structural MRI | Original PET image | Recovery coefficients | PET after regional PVE correction |

Fig. 2. Structural MRI is used to segment the PET image and calculate the recovery coefficients for partial volume effect (PVE) correction. MRI and PET data were acquired simultaneously on the BrainPET prototype, Martinos Center at Massachusetts General Hospital. (This research was originally published in *JNM*. Catana C, Drzezga A. PET/MRI for neurological applications. J Nucl Med 2012;53(12):1918. © by the Society of Nuclear Medicine and Molecular Imaging, Inc.)

systems. On combined PET–MRI systems, there is also an opportunity to exploit motion correction techniques already developed for MRI to correct the temporally and spatially registered PET data. This correction is performed simply by applying the transformation matrix determined for MR image correction to the PET images.[41] Different motion correction methods are available depending on the motion type, that is, rigid body motion only or nonrigid body motion.

Rigid Body Motion Correction

Rigid body motion correction is used to correct for (1) rapid head movements such as those experienced by patients with Tourette syndrome or Parkinson's disease and (2) the slow drift of the head induced by muscle relaxation during long scans. Thus, an effective motion correction scheme must have a high temporal resolution to correct for rapid movements as well as a high sensitivity to detect gradual head shift. A simple image-based technique for rigid motion correction consists in acquiring full images at different time frames and registering each one to a reference frame.[42] However, the temporal resolution of common acquisition schemes designed to cover an extended body area may not be sufficient to correct for rapid motion. Using a fast sequence, such as EPI with a temporal resolution of 2 to 3 seconds, was found to improve image quality significantly (eg, reduced blurring or artifacts)[43] and time–activity curves estimation.[44] However, EPI cannot track very fast motion.

If a greater temporal resolution is required or if concomitant anatomic, rather than functional, MRI is desired, navigator echoes such as cloverleaf navigators[45] are an option. These 20-ms acquisitions provide a reference for motion correction and can be integrated in any steady-state 3D sequence, with workarounds possible for other sequence types. However, cloverleaf navigators do not provide adequate motion correction in the case of large movements (>10 mm or >10°).[43]

Nonrigid Body Motion Correction

Correcting for cardiac and respiratory motion requires nonrigid image registration, which takes into account complex motion fields induced by the deformation of numerous tissues as well as intracyclic and intercyclic variability. In the early days of PET–MRI, proof-of-concept nonrigid motion correction was performed using series of structural MR images of slow-moving phantoms.[46] Afterward, fast sequences based on keyhole and parallel imaging have been tested in simulations,[47] and improvement was noted for motion corrected PET images in regions of high MRI contrast. For regions of low contrast, an option is to use RF tagging to superimpose a periodic pattern on anatomic features and to quantify its deformation (**Fig. 3**).[48–51] Note that tagging cannot be used in regions with very low signal, such as the lungs,[48] and is hard to implement for respiratory motion in humans because the pattern fades away quickly.[52] Computing motion fields for the whole cardiac and respiratory cycle with the previous methods require

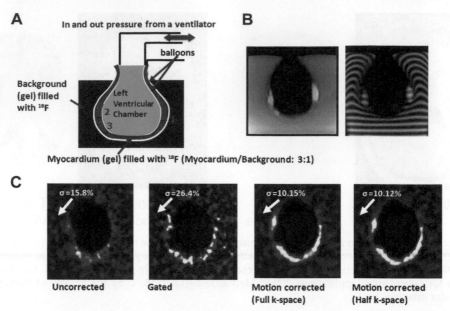

Fig. 3. (*A*) Cardiac phantom used to assess PET motion correction based on MRI tagging in a bimodal PET–MRI system. (*B*) Untagged and tagged MR images. (*C*) PET images without correction, with gating and with motion correction. Half k-space reduces MRI acquisition time for the purpose of motion correction from 12 minutes to less than 5 minutes. (*From* Ouyang J, Li Q, El Fakhri G. Magnetic resonance-based motion correction for positron emission tomography imaging. Semin Nucl Med 2013;43(1):64; with permission.)

gating of the data using either external devices or the images themselves. This latter method, known as self-gating, has been implemented using the profiles of a radial acquisition[53] or navigator echoes[41,52,54] to track an anatomic feature such as the liver or the diaphragm.

Acquiring image series or tagging patterns solely for the purpose of motion correction can limit the types of concurrent MRI sequences performed during the PET scan. As a workaround for abdominal imaging, it is possible to use a model of the respiratory cycle specific to each patient. The model is developed by acquiring images of the whole respiratory cycle at the beginning of the PET scan. Afterward, each PET time frame is registered to this model using navigator echoes.[52,54] Other MRI sequences can then be acquired during the PET scan after the model has been built as long as it is possible to include the navigator echoes in these sequences. However, model-based motion correction cannot explicitly account for intracyle or intercycle variations. King and colleagues[55] suggested a principal component analysis method which incorporates a 3D dynamic model and 2D MR image navigator to account for these variations, but it requires parallel imaging with state-of-the-art multichannel coils that are not available on all systems.

MR Active Markers

MR active markers (coils that can be tracked with a special pulse sequence) are another avenue in MRI motion correction that can be applied to PET images acquired simultaneously. Both wired and wireless markers have been tested successfully[56,57] in clinical and preclinical studies. These markers are tracked at short intervals (around 50 ms) by a dedicated pulse sequence, lasting about 10 ms, that can be incorporated in most 2D and 3D imaging routines, with the exception of certain steady-state free precession sequences.[57] These markers have been tracked efficiently over a range of 45 mm and 20° in regions of gradient linearity and can thus be useful for the correction of large movements.[56] MR active markers are also noted for their versatility: they can be used for rigid motion correction[57] and for thoracic or intracavity nonrigid motion correction of small regions; however, surrounding regions may suffer from enhanced artifacts.[56]

Computational Aspect of Motion Correction

Motion correction can be performed after or during image reconstruction. Postreconstruction motion correction is achieved by reconstructing many short time frames relatively devoid of motion artifacts and registering them. Once the frames are properly registered, they can be summed up to retrieve low temporal resolution frames with higher signal, producing a clearer image of the tracer distribution in the ROI. No modification of the reconstruction process is required. However, this approach reduces the signal-to-noise ratio because of the limited count statistics for each time frame during the reconstruction.[44] Reconstructing many short time frames is also more computer intensive than reconstructing a single volume. When motion information is integrated in the line of response space, count statistics are preserved and the motion can be approximated by a continuous function, allowing the user to select the duration of each time frame.[54] Moreover, the line of response motion correction process takes only a small part of the overall reconstruction process.[44] For these reasons, motion correction usually proves faster when implemented as part of the reconstruction process. In all cases, the computing time can be reduced by using parallelization or by setting a threshold (in degrees or mm) under which motion is not corrected.[43]

PET–MRI ARTERIAL INPUT FUNCTION CONVERSION

In a preclinical setting, efforts were recently made to deduce the AIF of a PET tracer from the AIF of an MRI contrast agent injected during the same study. The technique has the potential to obviate the need for PET data in the process of obtaining the PET tracer AIF. Indeed, it was shown that the pharmacokinetic parameters obtained with the converted Gd-DTPA AIF are similar to those obtained with the fluorodeoxyglucose or the [^{18}F]fluoroethyl-L-tyrosine AIFs.[4,58] These studies on AIF conversion have been conducted using both blood- and image-derived Gd-DTPA AIF and both methods proved valid.[4,59] For instance, Poulin and colleagues[4] derived the MRI AIF from an RR, a method that requires only the MR images, a priori information on the tissue kinetics, and a simple set of conversion rules specific to the MRI contrast agent (Gd-DTPA) and the PET tracer (fluorodeoxyglucose). Evans and colleagues[60] have also shown that it is possible to automatically detect the first pass bolus of a gadolinium-based agent in EPI images of rat brains. This automatic detection of a blood signal allows direct IDAIF extraction without the need for a well-characterized tissue of reference. Finally, work has been undertaken to transpose the AIF conversion technique to a clinical setting,[3] but the bias it could induce still needs further evaluation.

CAVEATS

The idea of deriving an AIF without arterial cannulation is appealing both to the clinician and to the patient. As outlined previously, the synergy of MRI and PET can improve the quality of the PET IDAIF through better segmentation as well as PVE and motion correction. However, each postprocessing step must be approached carefully because it can introduce errors owing to misregistration, missegmentation, or imperfect correction. Even in the case of simultaneous PET–MRI, the temporal and spatial registration of both modalities must be calibrated carefully.[43]

The nature of the radiotracer can also limit the possibility of deriving the AIF solely from images, notably in the presence of radiometabolites.[61,62] Discriminating radiometabolites and the parent radiotracer is problematic when deriving the AIF from blood pools. Results obtained after calibration of the IDAIF with a limited number of arterial blood samples are closer to those observed with a blood AIF, but only for compounds producing few radiometabolites.[61,63,64] Compounds rapidly metabolized in blood generating many radiometabolites remain problematic.[61] Late venous samples or average radiometabolite curves can be substituted for arterial samples in some cases[22,63,65] and could be used to calibrate the IDAIF without arterial cannulation; this option must be validated for each probe.

Image-derived AIF substitutes outperform blood AIFs in some cases. For example, it has been shown that using a simplified reference tissue model[66] to estimate the binding potential of some probes in brain regions is more robust than relying on blood AIF. This demonstration has been made for probes that have very fast, or very slow, plasma clearance[67,68] making it difficult to fit the concentration curve to a specific kinetic model. Other reference tissue methods such as the multilinear reference tissue model have produced robust results as well.[69] A decrease in intersubject variability was also observed in the case of cerebral blood flow estimation by [^{15}O]-water PET when using an IDAIF rather than the AIF derived from blood samples. To explain this result, Fung and colleagues[13] postulated that the carotid arteries would be more representative of the local brain AIF compared with the AIF derived by sampling from the radial artery, even after correction for dispersion. Indeed, the correction factor for dispersion applied to the blood AIF is usually the same for all subjects, whereas hemodynamic parameters can vary significantly between individuals.

SUMMARY

Although it may not be possible to eliminate arterial blood sampling completely from all quantitative PET protocols, an appropriate IDAIF or an AIF conversion method can reduce the number of blood samples required and, therefore, the workload associated with these studies. Also, the IDAIF may be more representative of the tracer concentration in local arteries and could outperform the blood AIF in some cases. It is possible to derive a more precise IDAIF, and therefore improve PET kinetic modeling, by leveraging the synergy of PET (straightforward measurement of a variety of biomarkers) and MRI (high-quality anatomic images, measurement of many physiologic processes, including blood flow, and adaptable pulse sequences). As shown previously, many developments in MRI-based segmentation, partial volume correction, and motion correction can be applied to PET images after image registration. In a properly calibrated simultaneous PET–MRI system, nearly perfect spatial and temporal registration can be achieved. On these systems, MRI-guided image correction can be performed easily without sacrificing other diagnostic MRI sequences. Therefore, this truly simultaneous quantitative imaging tool has the potential to improve diagnosis precision significantly while decreasing the length and number of examinations for the patient.

REFERENCES

1. Gambhir SS, Schwaiger M, Huang SC, et al. Simple noninvasive quantification method for measuring myocardial glucose utilization in humans employing positron emission tomography and fluorine-18 deoxyglucose. J Nucl Med 1989;30(3):359–66.
2. Su Y, Arbelaez AM, Benzinger TLS, et al. Noninvasive estimation of the arterial input function in positron emission tomography imaging of cerebral blood flow. J Cereb Blood Flow Metab 2013;33(1):115–21.
3. Sari H, Erlandsson K, Barnes A, et al. Modelling the impact of injection time on the bolus shapes in PET-MRI AIF conversion. EJNMMI Phys 2014; 1(Suppl 1):A54.
4. Poulin E, Lebel R, Croteau E, et al. Conversion of arterial input functions for dual pharmacokinetic modeling using Gd-DTPA/MRI and 18F-FDG/PET. Magn Reson Med 2013;69(3):781–92.
5. Da Silva NA, Herzog H, Weirich C, et al. Image-derived input function obtained in a 3TMR-brainPET. Nucl Instrum Methods Phys Res A 2012;702:22–5.
6. Chen K, Bandy D, Reiman E, et al. Noninvasive quantification of the cerebral metabolic rate for glucose using positron emission tomography, 18F-fluoro-2-deoxyglucose, the Patlak method, and an image-derived input function. J Cereb Blood Flow Metab 1998;18(7):716–23.
7. Lammertsma AA, Bench CJ, Hume SP, et al. Comparison of methods for analysis of clinical [11C]raclopride studies. J Cereb Blood Flow Metab 1996;16(1):42–52.
8. Gutierrez D, Montandon M-L, Assal F, et al. Anatomically guided voxel-based partial volume effect correction in brain PET: impact of MRI segmentation. Comput Med Imaging Graph 2012; 36(8):610–9.
9. Fung EK, Planeta-Wilson B, Mulnix T, et al. A multimodal approach to image-derived input functions for brain PET. IEEE Nucl Sci Symp Conf Rec (1997) 2009;2009:2710–4.
10. Müllor Gärtner HW, Links JM, Prince JL, et al. Measurement of radiotracer concentration in brain gray matter using positron emission tomography: MRI-based correction for partial volume effects. J Cereb Blood Flow Metab 1992;12(4):571–83.
11. Shan ZY, Mateja SJ, Reddick WE, et al. Retrospective evaluation of PET-MRI registration algorithms. J Digit Imaging 2011;24(3):485–93.
12. Kiebel S, Ashburner J, Poline J, et al. MRI and PET coregistration — a cross validation of statistical parametric mapping and automated image registration. Neuroimage 1997;5(4 pt 1):271–9.
13. Fung E, Carson R. Cerebral blood flow with [15O]-water PET studies using an image-derived input function and MR-defined carotid centerlines. Phys Med Biol 2013;58(6):1903–23.
14. Nekolla SG, Martinez-Moeller A, Saraste A. PET and MRI in cardiac imaging: from validation studies to integrated applications. Eur J Nucl Med Mol Imaging 2009;36(Suppl 1):S121–30.
15. Yankeelov TE, Peterson TE, Abramson RG, et al. Simultaneous PET-MRI in oncology: a solution looking for a problem? Magn Reson Imaging 2012; 30(9):1342–56.
16. Rakheja R, DeMello L, Chandarana H, et al. Comparison of the accuracy of PET/CT and PET/MRI spatial registration of multiple metastatic lesions. Am J Roentgenol 2013;201(5):1120–3.
17. Gordillo N, Montseny E, Sobrevilla P. State of the art survey on MRI brain tumor segmentation. Magn Reson Imaging 2013;31(8):1426–38.
18. Bauer S, Wiest R, Nolte L-P, et al. A survey of MRI-based medical image analysis for brain tumor studies. Phys Med Biol 2013;58(13):R97–129.
19. Cabezas M, Oliver A, Lladó X, et al. A review of atlas-based segmentation for magnetic resonance brain images. Comput Methods Programs Biomed 2011;104(3):e158–77.
20. Wong K-P, Feng D, Meikle SR, et al. Segmentation of dynamic PET images using cluster analysis. IEEE Trans Nucl Sci 2002;49(1):200–7.

21. Turkheimer FE, Edison P, Pavese N, et al. Reference and target region modeling of [11C]-(R)-PK11195 brain studies. J Nucl Med 2007;48(1):158–67.

22. Rissanen E, Tuisku J, Luoto P, et al. Automated reference region extraction and population-based input function for brain [11C]TMSX PET image analyses. J Cereb Blood Flow Metab 2015;35(1):157–65.

23. Lyoo CH, Zanotti-Fregonara P, Zoghbi SS, et al. Image-derived input function derived from a supervised clustering algorithm: methodology and validation in a clinical protocol using [11C](R)-rolipram. PLoS One 2014;9(2):e89101.

24. Iguchi S, Hori Y, Moriguchi T, et al. Verification of a semi-automated MRI-guided technique for non-invasive determination of the arterial input function in15O-labeled gaseous PET. Nucl Instrum Methods Phys Res A 2013;702:111–3.

25. Surti S, Shore AR, Karp JS. Design study of a whole-body PET scanner with improved spatial and timing resolution. IEEE Trans Nucl Sci 2013;60(5): 3220–6.

26. Virdee K, Cumming P, Caprioli D, et al. Applications of positron emission tomography in animal models of neurological and neuropsychiatric disorders. Neurosci Biobehav Rev 2012;36(4):1188–216.

27. Moses WW. Fundamental limits of spatial resolution in PET. Nucl Instrum Methods Phys Res A 2011; 648:S236–40.

28. Catana C, Drzezga A. PET/MRI for neurologic applications. J Nucl Med 2012;53(12):1916–25.

29. Krejza J, Arkuszewski M, Kasner SE, et al. Carotid artery diameter in men and women and the relation to body and neck size. Stroke 2006;37(4): 1103–5.

30. Rousset OG, Deep P, Kuwabara H, et al. Effect of partial volume correction on estimates of the influx and cerebral metabolism of 6-[18 F] fluoro-L-dopa studied with PET in normal control and Parkinson's disease subjects. Synapse 2000;37(2):81–9.

31. Videen TO, Perlmutter JS, Mintun MA, et al. Regional correction of positron emission tomography data for the effects of cerebral atrophy. J Cereb Blood Flow Metab 1988;8(5):662–70.

32. Meltzer C, Kinahan P, Greer P, et al. Comparative evaluation of MR-based partial-volume correction schemes for PET. J Nucl Med 1999;40(12):2053–65.

33. Rousset OG, Ma Y, Evans AC. Correction for partial volume effects in PET: principle and validation. J Nucl Med 1998;39(5):904–11.

34. Boussion N, Hatt M, Lamare F, et al. A multiresolution image based approach for correction of partial volume effects in emission tomography. Phys Med Biol 2006;51(7):1857–76.

35. Shidahara M, Tsoumpas C, Hammers A, et al. Functional and structural synergy for resolution recovery and partial volume correction in brain PET. Neuroimage 2009;44(2):340–8.

36. Le Pogam A, Hatt M, Descourt P, et al. Evaluation of a 3D local multiresolution algorithm for the correction of partial volume effects in positron emission tomography. Med Phys 2011;38(9):4920–33.

37. Le Pogam A, Lamare F, Hatt M, et al. MRI data driven partial volume effects correction in PET imaging using 3D local multi-resolution analysis. Nucl Instrum Methods Phys Res A 2013;702:39–41.

38. Mourik JEM, Lubberink M, Lammertsma AA, et al. Image derived input functions: effects of motion on tracer kinetic analyses. Mol Imaging Biol 2011; 13(1):25–31.

39. Lamare F, Le Maitre A, Dawood M, et al. Evaluation of respiratory and cardiac motion correction schemes in dual gated PET/CT cardiac imaging. Med Phys 2014; 41(2014):072504.

40. Fulton RR, Meikle SR, Eberl S, et al. Correction for head movements in positron emission tomography using an optical motion-tracking system. IEEE Trans Nucl Sci 2002;49(1):116–23.

41. Ouyang J, Li Q, El Fakhri G. Magnetic resonance-based motion correction for positron emission tomography imaging. Semin Nucl Med 2013;43(1):60–7.

42. Picard Y, Thompson CJ. Motion correction of PET images using multiple acquisition frames. IEEE Trans Med Imaging 1997;16(2):137–44.

43. Catana C, Benner T, van der Kouwe A, et al. MRI-assisted PET motion correction for neurologic studies in an integrated MR-PET scanner. J Nucl Med 2011;52(1):154–61.

44. Ullisch MG, Scheins JJ, Weirich C, et al. MR-based PET motion correction procedure for simultaneous MR-PET neuroimaging of human brain. PLoS One 2012;7(11):e48149.

45. Van der Kouwe AJW, Benner T, Dale AM. Real-time rigid body motion correction and shimming using cloverleaf navigators. Magn Reson Med 2006; 56(5):1019–32.

46. Tsoumpas C, Mackewn JE, Halsted P, et al. Simultaneous PET-MR acquisition and MR-derived motion fields for correction of non-rigid motion in PET. Ann Nucl Med 2010;24(10):745–50.

47. Dikaios N, Izquierdo-Garcia D, Graves MJ, et al. MRI-based motion correction of thoracic PET: initial comparison of acquisition protocols and correction strategies suitable for simultaneous PET/MRI systems. Eur Radiol 2012;22(2):439–46.

48. Guérin B, Cho S, Chun SY, et al. Nonrigid PET motion compensation in the lower abdomen using simultaneous tagged-MRI and PET imaging. Med Phys 2011;38(6):3025.

49. Chun SY, Reese TG, Ouyang J, et al. MRI-based nonrigid motion correction in simultaneous PET/MRI. J Nucl Med 2012;53(8):1284–91.

50. Fieseler M, Kugel H, Gigengack F, et al. A dynamic thorax phantom for the assessment of cardiac and respiratory motion correction in PET/MRI: a

preliminary evaluation. Nucl Instrum Methods Phys Res A 2013;702:59–63.

51. Petibon Y, Ouyang J, Zhu X, et al. Cardiac motion compensation and resolution modeling in simultaneous PET-MR: a cardiac lesion detection study. Phys Med Biol 2013;58(7):2085–102.

52. Petibon Y, Huang C, Ouyang J, et al. Relative role of motion and PSF compensation in whole-body oncologic PET-MR imaging. Med Phys 2014;41(4): 042503.

53. Grimm R, Sebastian F, Dregely I, et al. MR-PET respiration compensation using self-gated motion modeling. Proc Intl Soc Mag Reson Med 2013; 21(2013):0829.

54. Würslin C, Schmidt H, Martirosian P, et al. Respiratory motion correction in oncologic PET using T1-weighted MR imaging on a simultaneous whole-body PET/MR system. J Nucl Med 2013;54(3):464–71.

55. King AP, Buerger C, Tsoumpas C, et al. Thoracic respiratory motion estimation from MRI using a statistical model and a 2-D image navigator. Med Image Anal 2012;16(1):252–64.

56. Qin L, Schmidt EJ, Tse ZTH, et al. Prospective motion correction using tracking coils. Magn Reson Med 2013;69(3):749–59.

57. Huang C, Ackerman JL, Petibon Y, et al. Motion compensation for brain PET imaging using wireless MR active markers in simultaneous PET-MR: phantom and non-human primate studies. Neuroimage 2014;91:129–37.

58. Fouquet JP, Lebel R, Lepage M. Study of the link between arterial input functions of FET-PET and Gd-DTPA-MRI for pharmacokinetic modeling. PSMR 2013. Aachen (Germany), May 6–7, 2013. p. 11.

59. Poulin E, Lebel R, Croteau E, et al. Optimization of the reference region method for dual pharmacokinetic modeling using Gd-DTPA/MRI and (18) F-FDG/PET. Magn Reson Med 2015;73:740–8.

60. Evans E, Sawiak SJ, Carpenter TA. MRI-derived arterial input functions for PET kinetic modelling in rats. Nucl Instrum Methods Phys Res A 2012;702: 126–8.

61. Zanotti-Fregonara P, Liow J-S, Fujita M, et al. Image-derived input function for human brain using high-resolution PET imaging with [C](R)-rolipram and [C]PBR28. PLoS One 2011;6(2):e17056.

62. Zanotti-Fregonara P, Chen K, Liow J-S, et al. Image-derived input function for brain PET studies: many challenges and few opportunities. J Cereb Blood Flow Metab 2011;31(10):1986–98.

63. Zanotti-Fregonara P, Hines C, Zoghbi S. Population-based input function and image-derived input function for [11 C](R)-rolipram PET imaging: methodology, validation and application to the study of major depressive disorder. Neuroimage 2012; 63(3):1532–41.

64. Zanotti-fregonara P, Zoghbi SS, Liow J, et al. Kinetic analysis in human brain of [11C](R)-rolipram, a positron emission tomographic radioligand to image phosphodiesterase 4: a retest study and use of an image-derived input function. Neuroimage 2011;54(3):1903–9.

65. Zanotti-Fregonara P, Maroy R, Comtat C, et al. Comparison of 3 methods of automated internal carotid segmentation in human brain PET studies: application to the estimation of arterial input function. J Nucl Med 2009;50:461–7.

66. Lammertsma AA, Hume SP. Simplified reference tissue model for PET receptor studies. Neuroimage 1996;4(3 Pt 1):153–8.

67. Yaqub M, Boellaard R, van Berckel BNM, et al. Evaluation of tracer kinetic models for analysis of [18F]FDDNP studies. Mol Imaging Biol 2009;11(5): 322–33.

68. Yaqub M, Boellaard R, van Berckel BNM, et al. Quantification of dopamine transporter binding using [18F]FP-beta-CIT and positron emission tomography. J Cereb Blood Flow Metab 2007;27: 1397–406.

69. Miederer I, Ziegler SI, Liedtke C, et al. Kinetic modelling of [11C]flumazenil using data-driven methods. Eur J Nucl Med Mol Imaging 2009;36(4): 659–70.

Moving?

Make sure your subscription moves with you!

To notify us of your new address, find your **Clinics Account Number** (located on your mailing label above your name), and contact customer service at:

Email: journalscustomerservice-usa@elsevier.com

800-654-2452 (subscribers in the U.S. & Canada)
314-447-8871 (subscribers outside of the U.S. & Canada)

Fax number: 314-447-8029

Elsevier Health Sciences Division
Subscription Customer Service
3251 Riverport Lane
Maryland Heights, MO 63043

*To ensure uninterrupted delivery of your subscription, please notify us at least 4 weeks in advance of move.

Printed and bound by CPI Group (UK) Ltd, Croydon, CR0 4YY

03/10/2024

01040298-0002